A DIY Guide to Telemedicine for Clinicians

S.B. Bhattacharyya

A DIY Guide to
Telemedicine for Clinicians

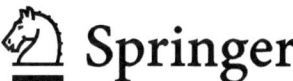 Springer

S.B. Bhattacharyya
Indian Medical Association
Haryana
India

ISBN 978-981-10-5304-7   ISBN 978-981-10-5305-4   (eBook)
DOI 10.1007/978-981-10-5305-4

Library of Congress Control Number: 2017955087

Printed on acid-free paper

This Springer imprint is published by Springer Nature
The registered company is Springer Nature Singapore Pte Ltd.
The registered company address is: 152 Beach Road, #21-01/04 Gateway East, Singapore 189721, Singapore

*In the loving memory of my dearly
departed father
Late Dipl. Ing. Santi Bhusan Bhattacharya
Respected grandfather (paternal)
Late Prof Mani Bhusan Bhattacharya,
MA (English)
And beloved grand uncle (paternal)
Late Prof Dr Bidhu Bhusan
Bhattacharya, MD
With all my love, care and affection*

Preface

At the early part of twenty-first century, the requirement of remaining connected to each other is no more a want; it is a need. Even though the maximum impact of this need is being felt through the ever-increasing use of social media, with the use of proper tools it will be in the healthcare domain where the maximum benefits are expected to accrue.

Before a collective groan emanates from clinicians the world over at this horrifying statement, let the author reassure all that things will become better and lives of clinicians much more worthwhile once this is adopted wholeheartedly lock, stock and barrel. Imagine a scenario where everything is interconnected to the extent that events can be predicted before they occur or at a very early stage. Preventive care, that holy grail of healthcare, will then have well and truly arrived.

The ability to predict the most likely prognosis from the temperature, pulse rate and blood pressure readings over a period of time in a sick patient in the intensive care unit can mean that an intensivist will be able to proactively intervene well before things get really desperate. A quick call to the nurse with immediate initiation of treatment can make the difference between a peaceful night and a hellish one. With the patient's relations aware of the criticality of the situation through better communication channels in real time, all stakeholders can be informed at every step of the latest developments regarding the patient's condition.

A sudden phone call in the middle of the night stresses everyone out. Knowing that things are bad and the future is critical helps prepare all both mentally and physically for every possible eventuality. This definitely will help deliver better care as the various stakeholders will then have had sufficient time to collect their thoughts and come up with the best possible solution, which might have a better outcome, as compared to one where they are left mostly to react to a rapidly developing (mostly deteriorating) situation.

Every time a patient makes a phone call to his doctor to ask for his advice and gets told to take some medication and then come and see him either during clinic hours or as soon as possible if things do not improve or get worse, telemedicine is at play. Yes, it is very low-end, but nevertheless it is telemedicine technology that has been used to provide immediate comfort and, most likely, relief. It is vital to note that *telemedicine is a technology and thus an enabler*. It enables providers to help provide more timely care that is better too.

Once all this is scaled up, the sky is literally the limit. The clinicians and patients can be co-located in the same dimensional space, albeit "virtually". With telemedicine, no patient is without access to his clinicians, most constantly, and a one-to-one attention can be provided to one and all – the holy grail of healthcare.

Too idealistic? Most certainly not, as we shall discover soon enough. Modern-day technology can make this a reality, costs notwithstanding.

This book attempts to help the reader to find plausible answers to the question, "How can I set up a telemedicine facility at my centre?" It does not however help provide the answer to "What is telemedicine and how can it be used in healthcare?"

The primary focus of this book is to guide the reader in using telemedicine technology to provide a level of care that increases customer satisfaction, which in turn increases revenues. Using the various methods mentioned in this book, the reader should be able to prepare a business case, formulate a business plan, cost the service mix and price it (including exploring the possibility of providing the service for free), for overall increased business volume. The reader should get a fair idea of all the tools that he will need for a particular service offering and where and how these might be sourced from. A word of caution is necessary here – since the tools are mostly IT and telecommunications-related, they are prone to rapid changes that result in newer and better offerings becoming available every few months.

A discussion on the various legal aspects is provided so that the readers are made aware of the various complexities and niceties that need to be taken care of and maintained at all times while providing telemedicine enabled services. No individual laws are discussed though as these vary from jurisdiction to jurisdiction. Needless to say that taking certain precautions and maintaining strict discipline will ensure that using telemedicine is a dream.

Readers will be well-advised to get their plans vetted by industry experts or consultants knowledgeable in this field to ensure that these are practical, or else they would most likely to be mightily disappointed when their bank manager refuses to grant them the necessary funding or the business venture goes belly-up. One cannot be too careful.

By providing guidelines that any clinician may use to set up and run a set of telemedicine services of his choosing, this book aims to facilitate a greater understanding of the technology and how it may best be harnessed to provide even better care. If some clinicians do begin to offer telemedicine services to their patients and the healthcare community is benefited by it, the primary intent of this book would have been satisfactorily accomplished.

The general approach of this book has been more of a minimalist in nature. Neither has everything been covered nor has any attempt been made to do so.

Haryana, India   S.B. Bhattacharyya

Disclaimer and Conventions Followed

Disclaimer

The author makes no representation, expressed or implied, as to the accuracy or complete-ness of the contents. These are based on his knowledge, understanding and experience that he has gained through his own medical practice and study of health informatics, including telemedicine technology, and represents his personal views and opinions.

The readers are therefore cautioned to use the information provided in the following pages purely as a basis for enhancing their understanding of the domain and then use their own judgement in using them. The author wishes to explicitly state that with the contents being purely a set of recommendations, *he will in no way be held responsible for the consequences arising from following them.*

The book contains a few imaginary case scenarios to help illustrate certain points. They are all fiction and any resemblance to real situations is purely coincidental and completely unintentional.

Conventions Followed

The various conventions that have been followed throughout the book are as follows:

1. The masculine includes the feminine, the singular and the plural.
2. The term "monitors" refers to both bedside and handheld monitors.
3. No specific application, commercial or free, has been described or named here as IT applications typically have a very short shelf life and are subject to very high turnover rates, thereby making a "hot item" of today an extremely "cold" one by tomorrow.
4. Generally for spellings, Indian English has been preferred.

Intended Audience and Chapter-Wise Outline

The primary intent of this book is to inform and guide the clinicians who wish to set up and run a telemedicine facility of their own. It does not intend to instruct, and the readers are strongly urged to refer to the authoritative body of knowledge that exists in the various subjects discussed. They are however free to use the contents of this book to act as triggers in igniting their imagination and then catalysing their interest in exploring the various options that telemedicine facilitates.

Although meant for clinicians, any care provider (individual or institution) will benefit from reading this book, and the term "clinicians" has been used to represent them as well.

The readers are requested to note here that "telemedicine" has been dealt with from two different perspectives: one, the technical side where telemedicine as a technology is the focus, and, two, the service side where telemedicine as a set of services is the focus. This seemingly contradictory approach has been necessitated due to the widely held perception that telemedicine is a form of medicine, which it is not. Nevertheless, this book primarily aims to guide, and in order to optimally accomplish that, it is necessary to use the underlying concepts as they are understood by the readers. Had this book been instructive in nature, the author would have attempted to convey the correct perspective, which is that it is a technology that significantly enables existing care delivery processes to "be with the times".

After discussing the history and definition of telemedicine, the term "digital health" is briefly addressed.

This is followed by a discussion of the general principles that need to be followed to set up a telemedicine service line. A section on social networking has been provided for the readers to have a broader understanding of this platform.

The next chapter deals with the various types of telemedicine offerings. Subsections in this chapter deals with the various types of services and centres that are possible.

This in turn is followed by a discussion on the infrastructural requirements for telemedicine.

Since telemedicine is a technology, an entire chapter has been devoted to discuss the various requirements from a technical standpoint and includes discussions on the various hardware, networking and software aspects. The various IT systems that help deliver better care have also been briefly dealt with. A subsection has been especially dedicated to the data vulnerability aspect, which is a matter of concern for all stakeholders.

Three different flavours of telemedicine services have been discussed in separate sections in some detail. The intent is to provide sufficient information to any clinician so that he may offer it to his patients.

The chapter following the above deals with the various management aspects. The pro forma I & E financial calculations of the three different types of telemedicine services mentioned in the preceding chapters, has been provided and the various aspects of change management and innovation diffusion have been discussed.

This is followed by a chapter discussing the various legal aspects involved with some recommendations for the readers to refer to.

A chapter on the concluding remarks, a glossary of many of the terms used, an index (of terms) and a list of references end the book.

A list of dos and don'ts, as home truths, has additionally been provided for quick reference purposes after the chapter on concluding remarks. This list is not telemedicine-specific and is more of an ethical nature.

The readers are requested to note that a number of items have been dealt with in the glossary section instead of in the chapters themselves. This has been deliberately done to ensure that the focus remains on the DIY aspects.

Overall Summary

Literally meaning "distance healing", telemedicine has largely failed to live up to its lofty promises of being a technology that transforms healthcare delivery.

In the following pages of this book, the author attempts to demonstrate how it can be easily adopted and offered to patients as part of their overall portfolio of services by the clinicians.

The author discusses the different flavours of telemedicine services that can be offered and the various aspects involved in adoption and offering them. The points dealt with include technology, service lines, guide to the methodology that can be adopted in setting up and running it, tops on the management aspects including tips on calculating the income and expenditure and pricing. Change management and legal aspects have also been briefly discussed.

The author hopes that the reader will be convinced that telemedicine can easily be adopted and offered to their patients without much ado at very affordable prices (the example I & E calculations for each of the suggested telemedicine service types amply demonstrate that this statement is indeed realistic). It will definitely be a worthwhile line of service to offer as it is bound to improve patient satisfaction by successfully addressing those aspects of healthcare delivery that are the root causes of most doctor-patient conflicts – lack of effective communication.

Acknowledgements

The author has heavily relied on the material from the capstone thesis that he wrote on telemedicine in the first-half of 1997 as part fulfilment of the requirements for his MBA in International Management. It was titled "Telemedicine: Information Technology—Its Place and Its Use".

He has also relied on the experience that he gathered during his efforts as a member of the National Taskforce for Telemedicine, under the aegis of the then Department of Information Technology, Ministry of Communication and IT, Government of India, in preparation and finalisation of the Recommendations on Guidelines and Standards for Telemedicine under the chairmanship of Mr B. S. Bedi, Senior Director of the aforementioned department.

He has also consulted a wide range of materials from various sources, including the Internet, which he would like to wholeheartedly acknowledge and freely admit.

The logos, wherever depicted/mentioned, belong to the respective copyright holders.

Faridabad, Haryana, India
April 2017

Contents

About the Author

S.B. Bhattacharyya is a practising family physician and health informatics professional. He studied in Medical College, Bengal (aka Calcutta Medical College), graduating with MBBS from Calcutta University in 1986, before completing his MBA studies in 1997 with a capstone thesis on telemedicine. In 2015 he was honoured with a Fellowship by College of General Practitioners.

Currently, he is member of the National EHR Standardisation Committee, MoH&FW, Government of India; Standing Committee of IT, Indian Medical Association Headquarters; and Healthcare Informatics Standards Committee, Bureau of Standards for India. In the past he has been Honorary State Secretary, Indian Medical Association Haryana State for 2015 IMA Year, and President, Indian Association for Medical Informatics for the 2010–2011 session.

Introduction

Ask anyone anyway associated with healthcare as to what principally ails it, the universal choice would fall on the *lack of communication between the doctor and his patient*. If communication is the problem, then telemedicine is the solution. By enabling the clinician to communicate with the patient $24 \times 7 \times 365$ irrespective of where one or the other is, it addresses this particular concern pretty effectively.

With the advent of the "connected" world, it is futile to resist the waves of change sweeping through all aspects of our daily lives. Naturally, the world of medicine cannot remain immune to this. The new mantra needs to be *"change or perish"*.

Telemedicine is such a vital part of the basket of care delivery services that it is already difficult and will soon be impossible for a clinician to continue to practise without using it. A technology and hence an enabler, by using it, any medical practitioner should ideally be able to *heal from a distance*, i.e. deliver care from a remote location. Using it, anything related to care delivery can be performed from a distance using this technology. Little wonder then that there appears to be *tele*-everything in care delivery these days.

There is a widespread perception that telemedicine and teleconsultation using videoconferencing or telepresence are one and the same thing. Nothing can be further from the truth. Telemedicine is not just about interacting with the patient like as if one were having a television show, with a studio-based anchor having a conversation with a location-based reporter to make everyone aware as to what all is happening out there. There is more to it than that, significantly much more. While we shall deal with the definition and various components of telemedicine in the next chapter, let us try and understand what exactly telemedicine needs to be.

Telemedicine as a technology enables any physical distance to become irrelevant to the provision of care. It neither makes nor aims to make a better clinician. Through its ability to connect the clinicians with their patients using modern-day best-of-available telecommunication and information technology, it facilitates the creation

© Springer Nature Singapore Pte Ltd. 2017
S.B. Bhattacharyya, *A DIY Guide to Telemedicine for Clinicians*,
DOI 10.1007/978-981-10-5305-4_1

of an ecosystem where they all may "virtually" exist in close proximity in the "cyber space".

Using telemedicine, a clinician should ideally be able to provide care to patients exactly as if they are "physically" next to each other even if they are miles apart. To accomplish this most effectively, it is additionally necessary that all the tools a clinician may require to provide the care are made available within the ecosystem in a manner where they can be meaningfully used.

Let us consider the following scenario. There is a medical doctor, let us call him Dr. Ex Why Zed, who practises as family physician catering to around 100 families located in and around his residence in a suburb of a metropolis spread over a large area.

At a particular point in time, he has four different patients admitted in three different establishments that are located in different places all over the suburb separated by distances of up to 50 kilometres. To attend a conference of vital importance to him, Dr. Zed has travelled to a place that is around 250 kilometres away.

Telemedicine will be able to help Dr. Zed to continue to care for all of his patients exactly as if he were not only still in town but appear to be physically present in front of them.

Medicine is an empirical science. To practise it, one needs observational data that is accessible on demand and occasionally on a need-to basis (not every physician needs every bit of data every time/all the time, e.g. a cardiologist will not need the power of prescribed lenses constantly be available to him, while conversely an ophthalmologist will not need the images of the last echocardiogram performed on the patient for every consultation). The sources of data are many, and with the advent of modern-day technology, such data get routinely generated on a continuous basis quite frequently. Technology now permits these data to be captured and forwarded over large geographical distances to all stakeholders in real time, thereby making it possible to treat patients from afar.

The role of the patient in telemedicine can neither be overstated nor overemphasised. In healthcare, the patient, and by extension the person, is at the centre of all activities of telemedicine too since he is the one who ultimately derives all the benefits that accrue, either directly or indirectly. A clinician with access to the latest patient data is able to consistently provide a better level of care to the patient. Thus, when planning for and selecting a particular set of telemedicine services, it is extremely important to constantly ask oneself, "How exactly is the person under my care going to benefit from this and to what extent?" It is vital to ensure that both "benefit" and "extent" are always maximal.

Telemedicine can, if properly used, enable clinicians to:

• Reduce overcrowding—use technology for triage to weed out the normal/those requiring attention that is either trivial or can be deferred for later— like, for example, middle-of-the-night inability to sleep, can be dealt with during regular clinic hours instead of as an emergency.

- Devote sufficient time to those who would benefit most.
- Use resources judiciously to maximise efficiency and outcomes.

The situation needs to change. To learn how clinicians can become effective "change agents" without much fuss, the author requests the readers to please read on.

Telemedicine

2

Abstract

This chapter deals with the history and definition of telemedicine, which is followed by a discussion on the newly and rapidly becoming fashionable term "digital health" that includes telemedicine as one of its main components (eHealth and mHealth being the other two). A section on the social media and another on social networking have been added to address aspects that are specific to them.

History

Ever since the spouse of a pre-historic man visited a pre-historic healer to report that her man was hot as fire while speaking deliriously and the healer sent her back with a concoction for her to feed him and inform if he does not become better, telemedicine is being practised.

Formed by the combining the Greek word "τελε" (tele which means "distance") and the Latin word *mederi* (which means "healing") to form the term "telemedicine" that literally translates into the phrase "distance healing". Readers will do well to note that the practice of telemedicine (and for that matter anything beginning with the word "tele") does not necessarily need computers. Any "technique"/"technology" that facilitates a clinician to deliver care to a patient is "telemedicine". However, to correctly appreciate telemedicine in all its glory, it is necessary to look at the evaluation of the technology through time.

Telemedicine, as we currently know it, began its journey when NASA concluded that the best way to continuously monitor the health of their astronauts from ground was to appropriately harness telecommunications technology and various health monitors. Needless to state, it was quite a resounding success. Encouraged by this, various medical institutions began running experiments of their own, for example,

© Springer Nature Singapore Pte Ltd. 2017
S.B. Bhattacharyya, *A DIY Guide to Telemedicine for Clinicians*,
DOI 10.1007/978-981-10-5305-4_2

5

Harvard Medical School set up a teleradiology referral centre in collaboration with Logan Airport. Results of the experiment were encouraging enough for other entities to conduct more ambitious ones.

This evolved into the concept of telemedicine as we know it today.

Definition[1]

WHO defines telemedicine as "the delivery of health care services, where distance is a critical factor, by all health care professionals using information and communication technologies for the exchange of valid information for diagnosis, treatment and prevention of disease and injuries, research and evaluation, and for the continuing education of health care providers, all in the interests of advancing the health of individuals and their communities".

It states that the following four elements are germane to telemedicine:

1. Its purpose is to provide clinical support.
2. It is intended to overcome geographical barriers, connecting users who are not in the same physical location.
3. It involves the use of various types of ICT.[2]
4. Its goal is to improve health outcomes.

The author however prefers the following definition that is simpler and easier to remember.

Telemedicine is the technology that permits delivery of care anytime anywhere to anyone irrespective of the physical location of the parties involved.

"Telehealth" is a new term that has since arrived on the scene. From a conceptual point of view however, this term "telehealth" subsumes the term "telemedicine", since medicine is a part of health. From a technological point of view, however, they are synonymous. In order to clarify, the term "telehealth" would normally refer to areas of preventive care and wellness management, thereby implying that it is more in line to serve the purposes as underlined by WHO's definition of health, which happens to be "a state of complete physical, mental, and social well-being and not merely the absence of disease or infirmity" as per its constitution adopted in 1948.

---

[1] The material for this section has mainly been sourced from Telemedicine: opportunities and developments in Member States: report on the second global survey on eHealth 2009 (Global Observatory for eHealth Series, 2). World Health Organization 2010 www.who.int/goe/publications/goe_telemedicine_2010.pdf.

[2] Information and Communications Technology.

Digital Health

"Digital health" is a new term that is increasingly being heard all over and rapidly catching the imagination of the concerned stakeholders. Simply put, it is an over-arching term that includes all aspects of IT-enabled healthcare like eHealth, mHealth, telemedicine, medical devices, biosensors, bio-monitors, etc.

While it has become fashionable to stick as prefix the letter 'e' to anything to indicate that the referred domain is "electronically enabled" and it is definitely debatable whether this is a good thing or bad, the practice itself does make sense. E-enabling a process definitely brings certain advantages to the stakeholders. For one, it makes things happen in quick succession regularly like clockwork, without exceptions, unless something happens to go wrong when the entire experience is likely to be more of a killjoy than anything else. Moreover, as the entire process life cycle is auditable, it becomes both transparent and optimisable.

These tools, like e-enabled monitors, IT systems, e-enabled mobile devices, etc., enable things to be done. The e-enablement of the care delivery process is what telemedicine accomplishes.

Telemedicine thus promises to make things happen not only from a distance but allows rapid intervention, almost on a one-to-one constant vigil basis even for non-critical care patients, while simultaneously ensuring that every step is audited and all deviations recorded for future reference, evaluation and process optimisation.

Medicine as a discipline exists because there are people with problems arising out of diseased conditions and state of unhealthiness when they get classified as patients. Once they become patients they need to be taken care of in a methodical scientific manner to ensure that their problems and diseased states are either eliminated in entirety or at least contained within manageable boundaries. Without the presence of a patient, there is no medicine to be practised. Now, a patient is a living, breathing, feeling being who is not at all happy with his condition—he is in torment, suffering. It is the job of the clinician to address the issues as effectively as possible to the patient's satisfaction—the higher the level the better.

Without continued access to the patient's past medical records, it is just not possible to provide the best of care. Thus, for any telemedicine encounter to take place, an EHR system containing information from the patient's medical past needs to be available on demand.

Therefore, as a minimum, the following four components are required for any telemedicine encounter:

1. Device(s) to generate data and interact (audio-visual) at the patient's end
2. Device(s) to display data/information and interact (audio-visual) at the clinician's end
3. Connectivity to link up the devices
4. Electronic health/medical record, preferably linked to the devices at the patient's end

Item numbers 1, 2 and 3 are mandatory. Item 4 is preferable but not mandatory and largely dependent on the needs and wants of the clinician. When item 4 is present, it should ideally be able to display the latest patient's clinically relevant information. This would mean that it is linked to the various devices that generate data at the patient's end and also recording the items of information that are exchanged between him and the attending clinician during any telemedicine encounter.

In the opinion of the author, having an EHR/EMR system is a great value addition. With all the various healthcare "things" (medical devices) and over-reliance on investigation reports, many gathered using monitors of all sorts, shapes and sizes; it goes without saying that it becomes necessary not only to view the data but also analyse the time series trends and past records to decide on what would be the most optimal course of action when tackling a clinical situation. To facilitate this, it is vital that one has continued access to an EHR/EMR system.

Based on the encounter context, the different devices will be needed at either end. However, an indicative list of the various devices would be as follows:

1. For interactive teleconsultation sessions:
   (a) Patient's end:
   - Video-enabled messaging app
   - Chat-enabled messaging app
   (b) Clinician's end:
   - Video-enabled messaging app
   - Chat-enabled messaging app
2. For a noninteractive telemonitoring/remote care sessions:
   (a) Patient's end:
   - Wearables
   - Biosensors
   - Monitors
   (b) Clinician's end:
   - Data display unit
   - Data analytics-based alerts and warnings system (remote care only)
3. For an interactive telemonitoring/remote care session
   (a) Patient's end:
   - Wearables
   - Biosensors
   - Monitors
   - Video-enabled messaging app
   - Chat-enabled messaging app
   (b) Clinician's end:
   - Data display unit
   - Data analytic-based alerts and warnings system (remote care only)
   - Video-enabled messaging app
   - Chat-enabled messaging app

Although somewhat over-simplistic as a list, it fairly outlines the various components that are generally required and mostly suffices. Some of these will be elaborated in later chapters.

Social Media and Networking

Telemedicine is considered to be that which takes place between a person seeking medical advice and a person dispensing that advice. A third person or a group thereof can be involved provided they can be classified as either carers or other clinicians. Thus, the use of any social media should not be considered as telemedicine. The following is provided here for information and due caution should be exercised when using this medium for any health-related interactions.

Social networking is conducted using social media comprising of websites and applications that enable users to create and share content with like-minded individuals for literally anything. Special purpose groups, like focus groups, can be created, and matters are posted for others to view and comment upon. All such posts are not one-to-one but are one-to-many instead. This creates its own set of privacy- and confidentiality-related issues.

Messages and the information they contain can be used and misused in a variety of ways with little or no control, and containment being only possible after the fact when most of the damage has already occurred. Privacy is severely compromised as every available content are open to public scrutiny of the most minute kind, both warranted and unwarranted. People have suffered severe emotional trauma for even their most innocuous of posts, with the occasional tragic consequences.

People using such vehicles for information dissemination would do well to remember that they should not post anything that they do not want the rest of the world to know, for the next moment may already be too late.

The author is of the opinion that the use of such mediums for any healthcare-related discussions, let alone telemedicine, is best avoided. The risks outweigh the accrued benefits by quite a distance.

Telepresence

A new solution introduced in the mid-2000s called "telepresence" has begun to replace the traditional videoconferencing. This is an experience that creates a feeling as if one is actually physically present at a remote location, using technology, even when in reality they are not. While popular applications are found in telepresence videoconferencing, technical advancements in mobile collaboration have also extended the capabilities of videoconferencing for the use with handheld mobile devices, making it possible to be present in the same cyberspace independent of location.

Needless to say, this is what is required for any telemedicine interaction of any type between various stakeholders (patient, clinicians, doctors, dentists, nurses, paramedics, care providers, professional colleagues, etc.).

3

Telemedicine Services

Abstract

This chapter discusses the various service types and their associated offerings that telemedicine technology can enable.

Overview

Physicians have long been advised to follow the motto—*primum non nocere* (first, do not harm)—and many have followed it most diligently. In not opting for a new technique or technology, this has been cited as the single-most important reason for repudiation—"Well, we hardly know anything about it, so better avoided till its efficacy is proven beyond any reasonable doubt", etc.

Noble sentiments for sure, but there is an important consideration here. Can one be absolutely certain that using it is more harmful than not?

Let us examine the following scenario to explore this question further. A patient is physically located far away and travelling from there is both arduous and expensive, possibly even hazardous, in his current condition. The need for travel is for a routine check-up by his doctor. The patient has been coming for these check-ups for quite a while now, and his test reports are all within normal limits. Now, there is the option for him to be able to get the review done using telepresence from within the confines of his home. He has a smartphone that permits video calling and his doctor has one too. For some reason, both of them have used the feature with others before and have found they can use them satisfactorily.

The dilemma now is whether the patient and his doctor should use the feature to conduct the routine check-up remotely or continue having physical face-to-face meetings as before. This is in full knowledge that it will certainly cost the patient's at least half-a-day's pay, apart from the travelling costs for an interaction that most likely to last no more than 5 minutes.

© Springer Nature Singapore Pte Ltd. 2017
S.B. Bhattacharyya, *A DIY Guide to Telemedicine for Clinicians*,
DOI 10.1007/978-981-10-5305-4_3

The most logical answer to such a scenario would be a definitive "no" and rightfully so. Thus, there is a pay-off. The dictum to be followed for all telemedicine services should be—is not offering the services safer and better than offering them? If yes, the services should not be offered. If no, they instead should.

There are a number of offerings that can be placed in the basket termed "telemedicine services". These include teleconsultation, telemonitoring and remote care.

At a very over-simplistic level, telemedicine is a sophisticated form of phone call with a little bit extra, where a whole lot more than just speaking and listening to the other end is carried out.

Service Types

Whenever anyone locates the term "telemedicine" the thought that immediately comes to mind is that it is an extension of the traditional clinical consultation where the interaction takes places using a glorified form of teleconsultation that is usually termed as "teleconsultation". This impression is erroneous for telemedicine is so much more than just that.

Let us try to understand why this is so and, more importantly, what exactly is telemedicine. The technology will enable any clinician (not just the doctor or the dentist but anyone who is responsible for providing care like the nurse, paramedic, nutritionist, physiotherapist, health worker, etc.) to be able to function exactly as if he is present right next to the patient irrespective of where the two are physically located in reality.

Consequently, what all will actually be required to use telemedicine depends on the exact nature of its use within the care encounter paradigm. This can range from using a messaging application at one end of the spectrum to a high-resolution TV quality audio-video communication at the other. Concomitant access to the patient's clinical records (in the form of EHR, EMR, radiodiagnostic images, investigation results and reports), monitoring devices (located bed side, critical care, home based, etc.), healthcare robotic systems, etc., may or may not be available.

Consultants of any healthcare speciality, ranging from general practice to super speciality like interventional cardiology or interventional neurology or radiation oncology or ophthalmology, etc., can successfully make use of telemedicine to ensure that their patients have access to them while they have access to the patient and his clinical data 24×7. As can be appreciated, this has the potential of providing optimal levels of patient satisfaction without tiring out the already over-exhausted clinician further.

It is extremely important to remember that telemedicine technology allows less qualified personnel to not feel abandoned or be at risk by having a friend, guide and philosopher available on demand to help out in case of need. This is especially required when having to deal with difficult-to-handle cases that require a level of competence that the attending physician does not possess.

The readers should note that the author has chosen to classify telemedicine services into six (6) distinct flavours as follows to help convey a clearer perspective regarding the functional areas that telemedicine technology enables.

1. Teleconsultation
2. Telemonitoring
3. Remote care
   (a) Telehomecare
   (b) Remote monitoring
4. Telesurgery
5. Tele-CME
6. Tele-critical care

Teleconsultation

Aka Virtual Consultations

This is what the be-all-and-end-all telemedicine is generally considered to be. Although it is not, the fact remains that most of the stakeholders consider it to be so. Consequently, it needs to be given its due importance in the general scheme of things.

Such uses are great for follow-up encounters but not so much for initial contact. There are some legal consequences that need to be borne in mind when conducting such consultations for the clinician (mostly) and the patient (occasionally). It is most unwise to treat a patient without thoroughly examining him first especially where a physical exam is crucial. Although haptics and VR might be able to address this aspect, nothing still beats the benefits of a real physical encounter conducted face to face.

The guiding philosophy normally applicable here is whether both the clinician (care provider) and the patient (person) are comfortable with the technology and willing to accept the consequences.

A legally valid informed consent needs to be communicated and accepted by the patient to the satisfaction of the provider before providing any such consultations. This is a must.

A further legal consideration has to do with licensing jurisdictions. Since the patient may be physically located in a geography where the clinician may not be licensed to practise, should the teleconsultation encounter be considered to be legally valid? The worries in this regard can partly be allayed by having a clinician who is licensed to practise where the patient is located to provide the consultation from afar or have someone who fulfils the criteria to be physically present with the patient who is the one who interacts with the remotely located clinician and then implement the instructions in the form of a set of orders of his own for which he assumes total legal responsibility. In the latter case, the consultant at the remote location acts as a referring physician and the provider with the patient as the primary.

In any case, it is wiser to seek legal advice to adopt the most legally appropriate process to ensure that all locally applicable laws are complied with. It must be remembered that ignorance is no defence in the eyes of law.

While payments for such consultations were an issue in the past, recently an increasing number of insurers are providing cover for them in several geographies (but not all).

Telemonitoring and Remote Care

Both telemonitoring and remote care work on the same principle (permit the clinician to continuously monitor and stay in touch with all patients under his care while providing care) and with the same aim (increase patient satisfaction and provide better care).

There are however some differences between them that are subtle but important. Telemonitoring is performed for admitted patients where the carers in the form of other care providers like nursing and paramedical staff, resident doctors, and visiting consultants, etc. participate in a harmonious manner to deliver care. A concert therefore needs to happen where all the stakeholders are connected together to ensure that the best of care is delivered at all times and proactive intervention can be initiated whenever any "early warning/danger signs" are observed. On the other hand, in remote care the patient is principally homebased or all on his own without continuous access to any carer, while his health is remotely monitored on a continuous basis and then necessary interventions initiated. This may be in the nature of an alert or a warning or a phone call to the patient or a visit by a care provider in the form of a nursing professional or a paramedic or a health worker making a house call on a priority basis.

Another important point of difference is that in remote care the actual monitoring is performed by a remote patient monitoring system. All the various health monitors and biosensors including wearables have their data either telemetered through to the remote system using various communications technologies or manually entered into the system by the patient or his carer, if he has one available. These are then processed in real time, and the corresponding alerts and warnings are triggered and sent across to the clinician (or any other designated care provider) for further action, which may be responding to a text message or a phone call or interacting with a care provider who makes a home visit in person.

Telehomecare

Aka Remote Patient Monitoring

The single-most important issue that complicates matters in this care setting is the fact that it is very difficult to control the space in the home-care setting since it belongs to the patient. While most equipments are miniaturised enough to be either worn or easily carried around by the patient, the "base" unit needs to be placed in a convenient place for it to be able to function optimally (mostly due to connectivity issues).

This means that such units (there may be several as one common base unit capable of handling all or many of the devices may usually be difficult to find) will need to be placed somewhere from where picking up the signals from the smaller devices and then passing them on can be easily accomplished.

These units will require 24×7 power supply and networking connectivity. Both Wi-Fi and Bluetooth® connectivity require continuous access to power supply—wired (regular power supply) or wireless (usually battery)—where even at low power consumption modes, they tend to continuously keep draining the batteries, which when old get discharged pretty fast. Furthermore, all such devices require regular servicing and maintenance. Fortunately, the more recently designed and developed ones need lesser attention.

Active-Assisted Living

Telehomecare differs from active-assisted living insofar as the former deals with only the healthcare aspects, whereas the latter deals with all aspects of day-to-day living that may or may not include healthcare aspects. An argument can certainly be made that "assisted" living is usually required by people who have healthcare issues. Thus, perhaps the difference is more about semantics, and it is better if the terms are considered to be conceptually synonymous.

Wellness Monitoring and Preventive Care

Aka Remote Person Monitoring

This telemedicine care setting definitely merits close attention. The principles at play at telehomecare equally apply to wellness and preventive monitoring. With many of the biosensors and monitors becoming wearables, IoT[1] is rapidly becoming almost the order of the day, with more stuff moving over to the "Cloud" for running, and mobile devices like tablets and smartphones almost becoming a part of the regular uniform of the common man, wellness monitoring and preventive care very much looks like the care offering that will transform healthcare like never before.

In this type of care setting, a normal person (or an ill one) will be able to have their health parameters monitored proactively to ensure that they adhere to a health regimen prepared in consultation of their physician or by themselves that will permit to maintain a healthy lifestyle and hopefully minimise, if not totally avoid, any health issues that may either be currently having or has the misfortune of developing in future.

The way the technology facilitates wellness monitoring and preventive care is discussed in the section on big data analytics in remote care later in the chapter.

Reimbursements by insurance are generally not available for any remote care, wellness and preventive care services, in most geographies for now. Telemonitoring may be reimbursed if it is done as part of a package for patients undergoing care in an inpatients care setting. This situation can be expected to change once such remote monitoring becomes more commonplace.

Role of Big Data Analytics in Remote Care[2]

At the outset, it is important to realise that not all data qualifies as "big data". Big data is data having some special characteristics. These are high volume, high

---

[1] Internet of things.

[2] www.asianhhm.com/information-technology/harnessing-big-data-analytics-deliver-optimal-care.

velocity, high variability and high veracity. In healthcare context, a good amount of data of various types from verifiable sources gets generated during a single patient encounter irrespective of the care setting (OPD, IPD, or emergency) even in a non-electronic environment at quite a reasonable rate.

With the use of electronic medical records (only), this amount increases dramatically as more data gets recorded and retained (volume). To this when the data collected by an individual gets added, the amount becomes pretty high. By 2015, it was estimated that an average US-based hospitals alone were generating 665 terabytes of patient data per year.[3]

Through the use of health monitors, medical devices and wearables, the rate at which the generated data gets collected is also quite significant (velocity). The types of this data ranges from binary to alphanumeric text including audio and visual, and in structured, semi-structured as well as unstructured formats (variety). The sources of these data are known and trusted with many being collected by those who have been authenticated prior to data collection like doctors, nurses, paramedics, etc. (veracity).

Coupled with the availability of large quantities of electronically processable data are a number of concomitant technical advances that is driving big data analytics. These advances include multicore processors, low-power-consuming devices, low storage costs overall and high-speed local networking.

It is the very nature of data that makes it qualify as big data, which makes their analysis demand special considerations. The process needs to factor in the high volumes of varied types of data in varied formats arriving very rapidly in real time. As a consequence, the traditional analytical processes are rendered impracticable, forcing special methods to be adopted to ensure that the analytics are carried out properly. Special systems for data storage, data retrieval, data preparation and data analytical are employed to ensure this.

Within the remote care paradigm, probably the most important benefit of big data and analytics is in real-time data processing and analytics, something that is almost impractical in other types of data analytics. The real-time aspect permits identification of the various indicators at an early stage. This leads to the generation of appropriate proactive warnings that in turn leads to early intervention. This helps in preventing more serious problems, averting crises and lessening morbidity and mortality, more frequently and sometimes considerably.

Data from the various monitoring devices at the patient's end get streamed into various processing systems where using techniques like signal processing, cluster analysis, pattern recognition, logistic regression, network analysis, etc., deviations from normal and potential problematic clinical states get identified rapidly in real time.

With the help of these alerts, the clinicians monitoring the patient are able to proactively intervene, thereby preventing health events, even stopping them before they occur or are able to cause any significant or long-lasting, let alone serious, harm.

The clinicians are able to get in touch with the patient/person and instruct them accordingly, e.g. asking them go visit a healthcare facility or go visiting them where

---

[3] www.aami.org/productspublications/pressreleasedetail.aspx?ItemNumber=1967.

they live (extremely useful in ageing population with chronic illnesses) or instructing them to carry certain tasks out, e.g. go lie down on bed or take some medication or avoid some food items, etc.

Big Data Analytics

Due to its very nature, performing big data analytics is not the same as performing regular data analytics. Since the data is voluminous, arriving at very rapid rates and of varied types, conventional methods of data analytics fail to be effective. While variety and volume can be handled, it is the rapidity of arrival (the velocity) that complicates matters. Such data cannot be efficiently handled using conventional Relational Database Management Systems (RDBMS). They need a distributed filing system like Hadoop Distributed File Systems (HDFS) for storing and a work distribution model that is able to perform tasks in parallel like MapReduce programming model for processing.[4]

While the mathematical models using in conventional data analytics are used for analysing big data too, since the methodology to carry out the calculations using models like MapReduce, these need to be suitably tweaked to function optimally. In models like MapReduce, the big data is first divided up (mapped) into different pieces that are then processed in parallel. The analytical results derived are then combined back (reduced) into a single result. Although the end-user will not (or hardly) notice any difference, the underlying processing is markedly different.

While using solutions like Hadoop will definitely prove useful in speeding up the algorithms processing of any analytics where data has large sizes (volume), it is necessary for analysing any data that arrives at a rapid rate (velocity).

Bottom line is that big data can only realistically be handled and analysed using IT systems that require considerable computing power.

Tele-CME

Applicable as for Tele-education/Tele-lecture for Healthcare
Telemedicine technology can excellently be used for distance training where live lectures, including surgeries, are broadcasted through to remote locations like medical colleges and medical conferences.

High-end lecture rooms and operating theatres/rooms are linked to specially constructed viewing halls capable of displaying surgeries being conducted and the procedure demonstrated by surgeons conducting the surgery.

The actual lectures and surgeries are beamed through using high-end video and audio equipment onto large high-resolution screens, and appropriate speakers are used so that the surgeons at one end are able to freely and meaningfully interact with

---

[4] Big Data for Dummies by Judith Hurwitz et al. John Wiley & Sons Inc.

the audiences at the other in real time. The lecturer/surgeon at one end interactively teaches and guides with the attendees at the other end.

Where surgical procedures are being demonstrated, special laparoscopes with cameras fitted to them are used. The images captured by these are then transmitted through to remote locations. Video cameras and audio equipment are set up at strategic locations in the operating theatres to pick up all the action and sound in sufficient details. These equipments help recreate for the audience at the other end the feeling of exactly what is happening in the theatre during the procedure, thereby conveying a realistic-enough atmosphere to them.

Equally, a highly experienced surgeon at the remote end can help instruct a less experienced surgeon at the patient's end to perform a demanding procedure proficiently with high levels of satisfactory outcome as a sort of hands-on training in procedures conducted from a distance.

Reimbursement is not an issue for tele-CME since no patient needs to pay for it.

The readers should note that the decision to stream live surgeries needs to be taken with due caution and after careful consideration. Patient-related privacy and confidentiality issues are at stake here. Bottom line, best avoided for conference settings. If conducted for training purposes, take appropriate consent—the language of which should be properly vetted by legal experts.

Telesurgery

Aka Robotic Surgery

As can be appreciated from the above section, it is possible to perform surgery, or for that matter literally any procedure, from a distance using telemedicine technology. The service is rightfully termed "telesurgery".

Here, the remotely located surgeon performs the surgery using a console that is used for visualising the field of operation while performing the surgery. The actual surgery is carried out at the patient's end by a robot accurately mimicking the actions performed on the console. As long as the connectivity between the surgeon at the console's end and the robot at the patient's end is present, it is a great tool in the hand of the modern-day surgeon.

Incidentally, telepresence technology is harnessed to provide tele-robotics, which telesurgery employs extensively.

Tele-critical Care

Aka Remote Critical Care

Here the various monitors and biosensors necessary to provide monitoring and care in critical care settings are telemetered through to remote locations. Since critical care requires these devices for continuously monitoring seriously ill patients, networking them to their "bases" located either at the nursing station or a room nearby with the intention of telemetering the data generated by them onward through to wherever they may be required is relatively easy.

Many commercially available tele-critical care solutions are already available in the market. By properly using them, intensivists and other critical care specialists are able to monitor patients under their care from remote locations, including the comfort of their home.

Infrastructural Requirements

4

Abstract

This chapter deals with the infrastructural requirements for offering the various types of telemedicine services. Only the clinician's end is considered here with the requirements at the patient's end being considered as being out of scope.

Overview

The telemedicine centre should be set up in appropriate surroundings that ensures the following[1]:

- Overall smooth functioning of the system.
- Patient's right to privacy.
- Does not cause interference to provision of telemedicine services due to external factors like light, sound, heat, dust, etc.
- Easy interaction between the patients and their clinicians.
- Power from standard electric supply or captive sources like invertors and generator sets or any other source is available during all telemedicine encounters throughout the encounter session.
- Proper connectivity between the patient and the clinician continuously established during throughout the encounter session.

---

[1] Adapted from "Recommendations On Guidelines, Standards & Practices For Telemedicine In India", Version 1.0, July 2006, Recommendations of National Taskforce on Telemedicine, constituted by an order of Ministry of Health & Family Welfare, Government of India.

© Springer Nature Singapore Pte Ltd. 2017   21
S.B. Bhattacharyya, *A DIY Guide to Telemedicine for Clinicians*,
DOI 10.1007/978-981-10-5305-4_4

Centres

When the equipment remains installed in a running condition at some fixed place, the centre is considered to be "static". Conversely, when the equipment is deployed on a mobility device or a trolley or on its own wheels (castors), the centre is considered to be "dynamic".

> *The currently-available gadgets makes centres to be more of a hybrid nature since some equipments would be fixed and the rest dynamic, with the number of equipments increasingly tending to be more dynamic than static.*

Static

Patient's End

The general room size should have sufficient space to accommodate the required equipments. The patient can be accommodated on a mechanised bed/chair permitting him to remain in one place/position, while the attending care providers/carers move around using the various telemedicine-enabled gadgets, monitors and devices as required. A conveniently placed single large screen that displays all information is better than having several smaller screens attached to each device to display the information generated by them. If necessary, the focus can be changed from one device to another to permit the remotely located clinician to view the necessary information correctly, although special software may be required to facilitate this.

Care should however be taken to position the screen in a manner such that the patient is generally shielded from anything that may potentially cause distress to him as he is unlikely to understand the full import of what all that is being viewed and may get anxious or even distressed. It must however be noted here that increasingly patients are not only becoming more aware about their rights and privileges leading them to demand to see the monitors as well. In such cases, the screen(s) will need to be placed such that they may be turned towards or away from the patients as necessary. *Do please note that to allow the patient to see or not is essentially a judgement call and almost always situational.*

For interacting with the remote clinician, the patient should not be required to make an effort to do so. Whenever any patient interaction is required, the audio-visual equipment (microphone, speakers, cameras and display screens) should all be conveniently placed for the patient so that the least amount of effort will be required of him to interact with ease. The fact that the patient is the focus of all activities at all times must never be lost sight of.

Clinician's End

A studio-like room is only warranted when the clinician is rendering teleconsultations. Adequate lighting with appropriate high-quality illumination that has adequate luminosity and sound proofing that generally blocks or cancels out all extraneous noises thereby making the provider both clearly visible and audible needs to be ensured. It is noteworthy that the equipments themselves may be a source of distracting noise, which may be consequent to their normal functioning or be generated in the course of using them, like moving them around. The room should be as stress-free as possible and to that end should be properly air conditioned.

The doctor's chambers, even if a single-room one, can double up as a telemedicine room without any changes. Need-to-have features will be same as above, while a nice-to-have feature would be sound-proofing.

Dynamic

Patient's End

Increasingly the various monitoring devices are becoming miniaturised, battery driven and lightweight enough to be worn on the patient's person or easily carried around by him with the least amount of inconvenience. The single biggest advantage of these equipments is that they are able to continuously monitor the patient 24×7. The downside to this miniaturisation however is that these need to be connected to some central hub using wireless protocols like ZigBee, Bluetooth and Wi-Fi or conform to Continua Alliance specifications.

Although the central hub could even be a smartphone, all connected devices, both mobile and fixed, need continuous access to both power and connectivity. The central hub itself needs to be connected to some remotely located central server or clinician, frequently in the Cloud, i.e. the Internet, which again requires 24×7 Internet connectivity and continuous power supply.

Clinician's End

When the clinician is at home or moving around or travelling, investment into such equipment that permits him to listen and visualise with sufficient clarity while enabling his voice and image to be equally well heard and seen at the patient's end will definitely be worthwhile.

Most currently available audio equipments (microphones and earphones) used in mobile- and home-based devices are usually well up to the mark in terms of noise cancelling, echo reduction and ability to pick up voices with excellent clarity as unobtrusively as possible.

Even if these equipments prove to be on the expensive side, the money spent is well worth it.

Virtual Hospitals

Perhaps that day is not far away when increasing number of people will be cared for in such facilities where the patients and their care providers will be co-located in cyberspace even when they physically are miles apart as population growth continues to outstrip concomitant growth of care professionals. In such facilities the patients may actually be in the confines of their homes and yet appear to be in an admitted facility complete with all the necessary equipments to care for them.

Alternatively, and perhaps more realistically, the patient may actually be admitted in a facility with the lowest possible number of care providers physically attending on him, while the rest are remotely located, perhaps in a central nursing station that serves as a mission control of sorts complete with all information available on large screens. The patient can be provided care round the clock where he can get in touch with any or all of his care providers literally at the touch of a button.

Virtual ICU
Several manufacturers are now offering these types of solutions that are geared towards critical care. The general principles remain the same as for virtual hospitals—allowing close monitoring of patients from a distance. The remotely located intensivists and critical care personnel are able to be "virtually" present at the nursing station or patient's bedside as necessary. This reduces reliance on telephonic conversations and feedback regarding such patients that require extremely close up-to-the-second monitoring and immediate care/intervention.

Using such systems, the intensivists are able to monitor patients under their care even from the comfort of their home or while in transit (travelling in between facilities and from and to their residence) and guide the nursing and paramedical staff, even relatively inexperienced residents, trainees and intensivists, to help achieve higher levels of care and consequent improved outcomes.

Virtual Wards
This is a recent but the most logical next step, following the introduction of virtual ICU mentioned above, with the concept of remote monitoring getting shifted from critical care to noncritical care settings. The best part of this is not the fact that the consultants, attending physicians and even the nursing and paramedical staff can keep a closer eye to the patients under their care. It is the fact that even the ward-based patients can have someone constantly monitoring them and be at their beck and call and with whom they can interact with on demand, albeit virtually. This increases patient satisfaction without impacting acuity while simultaneously assuring a handsome return on investment in providing the facility.

Home Based

The importance of homecare keeps on growing by the day without any signs of abatement. At the current rates soon enough, most care delivery is more likely to happen in homecare settings than not. While it may be useful to debate the pros and cons of delivering such type of care, the fact remains that it is already a reality and the entire healthcare community needs to accept this fact, making the necessary adjustments and business process re-engineering to make its adoption as painless as possible.

Homecare settings have its own positives and negatives. It is great for active assisted living but not so much for those who cherish their privacy. The underlying privacy concerns remain as the people who actually have access to the data remain unknown, and these continue to remain difficult to allay even with the best arguments. Especially since a lot of ghastly stories of data breach, being taken hostage through ransomware, not to mention the ever-lurking suspicion that some "nanny" is watching like a hawk in the form of overreach by various governmental agencies, both sanctioned and unsanctioned, keep popping up in the media almost on a daily basis. It is nevertheless interesting to note here that using technology, like in the form of end-to-end encryption, role-based access control with audit trail of every activity related to data management, it is possible to provide sufficient degrees of data security. Nevertheless, totally convincing the stakeholders continues to remain a considerable challenge.

Building (or Room)

Generally

> *The most important consideration should be that the telemedicine room is located in an easily accessible place for all the stakeholders.*

Dimensions

The minimum dimensions should be enough to physically accommodate all the stakeholders and the necessary equipment to support the telemedicine activity. It is generally the case that any room size less than $6' \times 6'$ (or ~2 m × 2 m) will likely be insufficient.

The room needs to be as noiseless as possible. For any stakeholder outside of a room, the use of earphones, preferably noise/echo-cancelling, is best along with a good microphone, preferably unidirectional, which are capable of picking up sounds as accurately as possible even in the noisiest of environments. For those behind closed doors, the use of good quality speakers and microphone generally proves sufficient. However, the use of noise/echo-cancelling earphones/headphones even inside the room is not a bad idea as the stakeholder can definitely pick up even subtle aural clues without much difficulty. The general argument against using earphones/headphones as they have a negative impact on hearing on long-term use continues to hold valid. The best course is to stop using them at regular intervals. A good way is to take periodic breaks after every telemedicine session.

The various equipments to be used for the telemedicine session need to be placed in an ergonomic manner. This means that if there is a large screen or a large equipment, these need to be placed such that they can be conveniently used even when moving around. Handheld equipments should be light enough to be comfortably held for long periods of time without tiring out the holder and additionally should have feather-touch response to be easy on sensitive fingertips.

The dimensions of the room/space are additionally dictated by the requirements of the video camera and the audio equipment used. Since the either parties are physically located at distant places and are able to see (and hear) only that what is beamed through, it is vital to ensure that they are both visible and audible to each other with as much clarity as possible. One of the key success factors for patient satisfaction is provider communication that is 60% visual and 40% aural. Even if the patient is not able to hear his doctor clearly, the ability to visualise him well enough is bound to have a favourable impression about the interaction. A smile being far more satisfying than a gentle word, a properly positioned video camera of sufficient resolution proves to be crucial for any telemedicine interaction.

It would not be out of place to mention here that as time goes by, the need for dedicated rooms is becoming largely redundant. Instead the need is getting restricted to a noise-free, well-lit environment with minimum of disruption.

Patient's End
The infrastructural requirements at the patient's end are dependent upon the patient's ambulation status along with the equipments necessary to monitor him plus those required by him, and his carers, to communicate with the clinician.

If the patient is fully ambulatory, then the monitors/sensors connected to him need to be portable, although not necessarily only wearables. The current networking protocols used to connect devices to their base units are sufficiently flexible to preclude the necessity of having to place them at near proximity to each other.

If the patient is partially or non-ambulatory and is largely confined to bed, then the equipment may even be fixed, or mobile and the audio-visual equipments need to be placed such as to ensure that he is able to communicate with the remote clinician in a manner satisfactory to both. The display screen and the speakers can be fixed or portable and need to be of sufficiently high resolution and fidelity. In cases where these need to be fixed for their proper functioning, the room or the place around the patient should be large enough to permit that.

Clinician's End
It does not matter where the clinician is physically located. He may be in a facility (clinic, hospital, etc.) or his vehicle (it is suggested that he should not be driving and either park his vehicle in a safe place first before conducting the activity or else engage a driver) or his home. The general requirements will not due to this.

Home Based
The infrastructural requirements depend upon the various monitors and devices necessary to provide telemedicine-based care optimally. While handheld or mobile equipments/apps require little no space, tabletop equipments will require appropriate furniture space to function. Consequently, sufficient space to house them will need to be available.

N.B.: Since this book is a DIY for clinicians, discussions on the patient's end are provided only to create awareness. Wherever it was deemed necessary by the author, limited details have been provided to facilitate clinicians to provide the services properly. Rest have been considered to be out-of-scope for this book.

Facility Based

Usually the room or space allocated to provide care in general proves to be adequate enough to provide care using telemedicine services. With Moore's law[2] in effect, the sizes of equipment and devices keep on getting smaller that have low power consumption, which may sufficiently be provided by batteries instead of requiring continuous high voltage power supply. This has resulted in lesser space requirements for optimal functioning.

Location

While the desire to be "far away from the maddening crowd" may sound sufficiently enticing to most, it is impractical in any healthcare setting since the "maddening crowd" is never ever "far away" enough. It is probably possible to ensure this at the patient's end, but less so at the clinician's end unless the clinician sets aside a certain amount of his time specifically for telemedicine on a daily basis or practises it from within the confines of either his car or home.

Irrespective of the telemedicine service being rendered, it is imperative to ensure that the environment be noiseless as practical as the patient rightly demands and most certainly deserves an exclusive one-to-one consultation with his doctor.

Where telemedicine is practised from a specially designed distraction-free room, the room should be located where an acceptable level of noiselessness exists—this "acceptable level" being determined by the requirements of the chosen audio-visual equipment and the general dictum being "the lesser the better".

For the patient receiving the services in his home, the location requirements remain largely the same—relative peace and quiet with adequate lighting cool environment and ample ventilation.

Where distractions cannot be totally eliminated, the aim should be "the lesser the distraction the better". Since the term "lesser" is a relative one, it should mean to be low enough to permit the stakeholder to provide his undivided attention with the minimal of efforts.

Access

In terms of physical access, the telemedicine room needs to have easy access, the considerations for priority access being secondary. This is true for both the clinician and the patient.

In terms of logical access represented by networking connectivity and/or access to applications, systems, monitors, devices and audio-visual equipment, both ease and priority-of access need to be given equal weightage with respect to importance.

---

[2] Based on observations made by Intel co-founder Gordon Moore in 1965, in its simplified version, it states that the processor speeds of computers or the overall processing power for computers will double every 2 years (http://www.mooreslaw.org/).

Miniaturisation of the hardware and low power consumption has meant that the need for allocation of dedicated space has become less of a factor.

Internal Fittings

It should be ensured that any cabling used does not cause any accidental hazard for people who may need to move around during a telemedicine session.

Ambience

Due to audio-visual requirements, the general ambience needs to be noise-free, with sufficient lighting at either end, as far as practical. The ambient temperature must be comfortable for all the stakeholders, wherever they are physically located.

> It goes without saying that the rooms, and preferably the corridors too, need to be air-conditioned with climate control. When providing care for one must be both physically and mentally relaxed and fully focussed.

Sound

Any careful evaluation of a patient requires the clinician to be able to listen to a number of sounds including those spoken by the patients and their carers, and produced by them, e.g. sounds from the heart, chest, abdomen, etc. This means that the immediate environment at either end needs to be as extraneous noise-free as possible.

Light

The ambient lighting needs to be of sufficient luminosity. Low lighting requires augmentation of visual signals through the use of low-light video cameras. Although many such image-intensifying cameras are available, even on smartphones and tablets, which are capable of generating a reasonably good visualisation at either end, there is no harm in having adequate levels of lighting.

Technological Requirements

5

Abstract

In this section a general overview is provided about each of the technical domains before discussing the actual equipments themselves. The readers of this book are not expected to be technologically savvy and the author felt that a general overview would provide a broader perspective and help put things into context. In the discussions where technical aspects are dealt with, the author has attempted to provide pointers that will help the readers to make an informed choice. They would nevertheless be well advised to talk to experts in the technical fields (hardware, networking and software) to procure and use the equipment that works best for the set of telemedicine services that they wish to offer. The author would however like to caution that most clinicians will find this chapter to be very challenging, in which case he wishes to inform them that no harm will come if they choose to give it all a miss.

Hardware

Like all other electronic devices, medical devices too have been following the Moore's law and becoming smaller, lightweight, more energy efficient and, best of all, more affordable. The golden rule universally applicable is that if a device can be connected to an onscreen monitor, it can be networked, and the same information can be displayed elsewhere without much difficulty, subject only to the constraints of connectivity and connection speeds.

Audio Visual

It is important to note that an encounter can take place without any audio-visual component being present where the clinician is merely checking up on the various patient records.

High-definition (HD) video cameras backed with concert-hall grade high-fidelity (hi-fi) audio equipments are used to provide as near realistic as practical an experience of being in the same "space" to all stakeholders.

With 3D and virtual reality backed with haptics, it may even soon be possible to "touch" and "feel". In short, the possibilities are endless.

As explained before, any communication has a larger non-verbal and smaller verbal component. This translates into assigning greater consideration to the visual aspects vis-à-vis audio. However, when any communication needs to take place, the verbal component must necessarily be available with the non-verbal considered as the optional extra. A verbal-only communication is always preferable over a visual-only communication. The reverse is not necessarily true.

Lighting that is unnecessarily harsh and uncomfortable should be avoided at all costs as these tend to tire the eyes out pretty quickly. The quality of cameras should be sufficient to render as realistic images as possible. The quality of microphones, speakers and headphones should be sufficient to recreate a feeling of a real physical encounter as close as possible.

Far-end camera control allows clinicians to take control of the patient-end camera and use pan-tilt-zoom (PTZ) functionality of the camera at that end. Even if there is someone like attending physician, nurse or carer present with the patient, this functionality makes it easier for the remotely located clinician to visualise the patient and his surroundings from various angles. The patient must be cautioned beforehand else the remote-controlled and automated camera manipulations themselves might cause him unnecessary stress even to the point of scaring him. *Incidentally, the patient too can use the same functionality to control the camera at the clinician's end. The author is however unsure as to how welcoming the clinician woule be of this functionality.*

It needs to be always borne in mind that the primary reason of all telemedicine interactions is provision of care. After all, the primary objective is to facilitate a telemedicine encounter, not put up a son-et-lumière show.

Display Screen

The opinion that display "the larger and the sharper the better" does not hold true for display screens and should instead be "one that is adequate" is a well-founded one for telemedicine. This naturally begs the question "what exactly is adequate?"

Any screen size that produces large enough images with high-definition (HD) clarity should be sufficient. There is a limit to visual acuity of the human eye beyond which no higher screen resolution will make much difference other than seriously denting the bank balance. Power consumption remains an important consideration, the lesser being the better.

It should however be noted here that where the digital solutions are used to analyse images, like for automation or artificial intelligence, for example, then the "more dots per inch the better" should be the dictum to follow.

Camera

A HD camera with enough pixel strength to render an image with sufficient clarity that fulfils the requirements of the corresponding display unit used at the other end is good enough. In short, the camera and the corresponding display must balance. Since it is not always possible to know the screen resolution at the other end, the safer option would be to assume that these will of the highest possible level, although perhaps not 4K.

While smartphone and tablet cameras come inbuilt and are easy to use, they usually have a very high quality one at the rear of the device and one of a lower quality at the front. Unfortunately, most telemedicine sessions make use of the front camera rather than the rear. It is therefore advisable to use a device that has HD-quality high megapixel camera in the front. The rear camera is not totally useless. These can be used to scan pictures and documents, which generally require better quality camera anyway.

For the patient's end, it is preferable that someone other than him holds the device so that the back camera can be used to take all images. For the clinician's end, the front camera is almost always to be used with the rear one for taking static pictures only occasionally.

Ear/Headphone

For audio, it is preferable for the clinician to use an earphone or a headphone irrespective of whether a laptop or desktop or handheld device is used. At the patient's end, the earphone or headphone is optional but preferable although may not always be practical since not only the patient but also his carers/care providers physically located by his side will need to listen in and respond.

There are three biggest advantages for using an earphone or a headphone:

1. These cut down the ambient noise and help deliver sounds with greater clarity.
2. The amount of radiation from the mobility devices tends to be reduced to the barest minimum.
3. It leaves the hands free to work instead of having to hold the device properly to hear the sounds.

There is a downside to using these for prolonged periods of time as sustained and regular use has the very distinct possibility of eventually leading to hearing loss. This can be partially mitigated by taking small breaks in between sessions from using them. An alternative could be using the speakerphone feature provided that the ambient noise is sufficiently low.

Microphones

Although the verbal part constitutes the lesser part of communication, by no means it is to be underestimated. A good microphone has much going for it to be recommended. Unidirectional microphones work better for one person, whereas multidirectional ones are better when there are several participants at that end. If the person speaking needs to move around, then a collar or tie microphone is quite unobtrusive and works quite well.

Incidentally, an earphone-microphone combination also works well for the handhelds including smartphones and tablets.

Speakers

A good-quality sound system that suitably renders the necessary sounds at a comfortable level—neither too loud nor too muted—to all the stakeholders usually suffices. There should neither be any echo nor hum as both are most irritating irrespective of the duration one is forced to suffer it.

Using PCs

These devices in the form of desktops, laptops, tablets and even smartphones come complete with inbuilt HD-quality web cameras and display screens, high-fidelity speakers and microphones, with provisions for connecting external cameras, speakers and microphone as well as extending the screen to an external one. These can be made very well use of, and using special applications, the devices can be turned into high-quality telepresence solutions. The communication link-up between two ends can be done using the Internet connection without any performance degradation. Several commercial products are available and it is definitely worth one's while to check them out.

Telepresence

This is a set of technologies that allow a person to get a sense of being on any location in the cyberspace, somewhat like virtual reality (VR) of sorts, even though the local (where one is physically located) and remote ends are in reality located at great distances apart. The control and feedback is accomplished by telemetering data and signals through cables, optical fibres, wireless links or the Internet. *Incidentally, when robots are deployed at the remote end and controlled from local end, this "telepresence" becomes "telerobotics".*

It does however demand a certain level of precision to ensure that the detection and perception at the remote end take place at an optimal level. This translates into the requirement that there needs to be exceptional image resolution, sound perception as well as haptics. Naturally, the volume of data exchanged are considerable, and to top it, it is absolutely necessary that there be no noticeable latency in mimicking the actions at the remote end. Problem is that no signal can travel faster than the speed of light. This means that if the locations are too far apart, there will inevitably be a certain degree of noticeable time lag. Thus, not only must the distances be limited but also the availability of large bandwidths is a must for this to work to everyone's satisfaction.

A very practical and most promising application of technology, especially in the context of telemedicine, is videoconferencing. This is probably the highest possible level of videoconferencing and involves using greater level of technical sophistication as well as providing improved fidelity of both video and audio than what is possible using traditional videoconferencing. Advancements in mobile technology have resulted in extending videoconferencing for use with handheld devices like smartphones and tablets, thereby making location-independent collaboration a reality. Consequently, the by-now-almost-ubiquitous smartphones or tablets and even laptops can be used for telemedicine sessions without much ado.

Incidentally, the term "telepresence" in this book has been used to refer to "telepresence videoconferencing" instead of "telerobotics".

Power Supply

Ensuring that there is steady and regular power supply is critical by some distance. The upside is that many of the equipments and devices use high-performance battery that only requires periodic charging. For those equipments that do not use battery as the primary source of power, power-surge proof uninterrupted power supply (UPS) systems are required to not only ensure that the equipment keeps on functioning during instances of power failure but also provide sufficient time to switch over to an alternate power source without any disruption.

> *A useful hack is to use a high capacity UPS system, much more than what the equipments that are connected to it require. E.g., if the equipment requires 100 W, use a UPS with not less than 1 KVA capacity. That way close to 8 times + the performance can be derived from the power supply source.*

Many wireless routers integrated with ADSL modems do not have any battery backup. To ensure that there is no loss of connectivity or downtime during instances of power failure, these need to be attached either to an uninterrupted power supply (UPS) or a generator, in which case a spike buster needs to be attached to ensure that no sudden power surges (which often occurs due to voltage fluctuations) damage the equipment while ensuring that there is no loss of connectivity. Although all UPS' have inbuilt spike busting capability, using an additional spike buster does a world of good since the many devices that use sophisticated electronics to run are very sensitive even to slight variations in power supply that are largely unnoticed by the human eye. Better safe than sorry.

Networking Routers

The most expensive equipment may not always be the best. A wireless router will provide more options besides eliminating the need to have thick LAN wires running all over the place and are usually preferred for connecting to the Internet or the Cloud. Incidentally, Bluetooth® or NFC devices do not need dedicated routers for connection.

Cloud Computing

This is a type of Internet-based computing. Here the Internet is used to deliver different types of computer-related services like server, storage, applications, etc., which are delivered to connected computers and devices. The various types of Cloud computing services are "software as a service" (SAAS), "platform as a service" (PAAS), "infrastructure as a service" (IAAS) and "mobile backend as a service" (MBaaS), and the deployment models are private, public and hybrid.

It should be noted that the term "Cloud" refers to the platform for distributed computing and the term "the Internet" the network of networks. The impression that "the Cloud" and "the Internet" are synonymous is wrong.

Incidentally, most of the Cloud-based EHR Systems mentioned in this book is more likely to be available as 'software as a service' than not.

Devices

Biosensors, Health Monitors, Implantable Medical Devices and Wearables

An ever-increasing number of healthcare-related devices are becoming available, with most of them being able to be connected via other devices that may use cloud computing to support telemedicine. These devices can broadly be categorised into two types—monitors and biosensors.

These devices are able to gather bio-signals related to vitals (blood pressure, both non-invasive and invasive; heart rate; respiration rate; temperature—surface and core), saturated partial pressure of oxygen, electrocardiograph, electroencephalograph, weight, etc. Multiple monitors, biosensors and wearables may frequently need to be attached to a single person to perform a wide range of health monitoring at any given moment in time. While some can perform a number of tasks using only one device, most of the time, several devices are required with each accomplishing only a single task.

Almost all wearables are connected using wireless technology, and usually the central (aggregating) hub is a smartphone, tablet or some similar mobility device. Many wearables periodically upload the collected data in an asynchronous mode, while others keep on continuously uploading synchronously in real time. This mostly depends on what the data collected by the wearables are to be used for. If it is for routine monitoring for future reference and evaluations, periodic uploading is the norm. On the other hand, if these are used as a part of active assisted living or monitoring those with chronic illnesses, continuous uploading is required.

With advancement in technology, most of the new non-wearable monitors and biosensors have wireless connectivity like Bluetooth® or Wi-Fi (some) or NFC that enable the data generated by them to be telemetered through to some aggregating device, which usually is an app installed in the smartphone. Although relatively expensive, the prices are now at affordable rates for many a pocket making them excellent equipment for telemedicine.

Handheld Devices

Smartphones, tablets and other personal device assistants (PDAs) are already powerful and are becoming even more so with nearly each passing day.

Almost close to a personal computer for all effective purposes in terms of computing power, storage and networking capability, these devices use GPS for location, accelerometer for motion, flashlight for light and sensors for proximity and temperature, capture and reproduce high-fidelity sound (through microphone and speakers) and capture and display HD or better-quality video (through camera and display screen). All of them additionally support a host of wireless connection protocols (Wi-Fi, Bluetooth®, NFC, etc.) that makes them able to receive and transmit data from external devices with compatible capabilities.

All of these features can be suitably harnessed to provide telemedicine services literally from the palm of one's hands.

Issues Related to Data Errors[1]

Since instruments in the form of devices are quite extensively used and the data generated by them are greatly depended upon to deliver care from a distance using telemedicine, it is important to recognise how data errors can creep in.

Out of the two categories of errors, namely, random and systematic, the latter can be avoided through methodical use with due care as these are mostly process-related errors of omission and commission resulting due to faulty devices, relative inexperience and carelessness like incorrectly inserting the leads or applying the device wrongly, wrongly reading and/or entering the results or, very rarely, due to instances of deliberate mislead (when someone wishes to "fudge" or "massage" the results to suit their nefarious purposes).

Although machine learning can help detecting the occurrence of such errors and factoring them in during data analysis, corrective measures need to be undertaken to ensure that the causes are identified and corrective measures taken (replacement of the device, end-user retraining, etc.) as soon as possible. While many devices have inbuilt safety mechanisms to alert users about the leads being disconnected or wrongly worn, wherever data is manually entered, there is every possibility of error creep to happen without anyone becoming aware that something is amiss for quite a while.

Issues Related to Radiation

There is always a lingering worry lurking around that all of these "electronic waves" created by the various gadgets like Wi-Fi routers, Bluetooth®, mobile telephone and

---

[1] This is not a discussion on the various types of errors like sampling and non-sampling (observational) errors, systematic and random.

the various devices that connect using them would not somehow endanger the lives of not only the critically ill patients but their clinicians as well, adherence to the various safety protocols, notices by manufacturers and expert opinion notwithstanding.

While it is virtually impossible to provide any categorical assurances, it is worthwhile to note that the dangers, potential or otherwise, are by and large offset by the benefits they bring. In all likelihood the radiation from cell phones is worse than that these gadgets emit.

Robots

Current (April 2017) medical robots are by and large confined to surgical care settings where they mimic the actions of the surgeon sitting at a terminal and performing the surgery using a monitor to visualise the part being operated upon. The actual surgery is performed by the robot (usually just a mechanised arm) on the patient. The robot is able to make the fine adjustments that facilitate for example performing cardiac surgery on a beating heart that appears perfectly still on the monitor that the surgeon uses, thereby eliminating the need for opening up the thorax and using a heart-lung machine while the heart is stopped. Of late, though, there have been several reports in various sections of the media of robots performing surgeries with greater degree of precision, thereby lessening tissue damage and loss of blood. However, these are yet to be commonplace.

Use in Telesurgery

Aka Telepresence Surgery

An early form of use of telemedicine in surgery, telepresence surgery is where the surgical consultant guides the surgeon, who actually performs the surgery, from afar. The remotely located consultant is able to be "present" during the surgery and visualise everything that the surgeon actually performing the surgery sees as well as interacts with the surgeon. This has facilitated in getting procedures carried out at higher success rates with less-experienced surgeons. The downside is the necessity of having a dedicated connection between the local end and remote end, apart from the need to have both the surgeries performed when the surgeons are at either end at their convenient time zones. The costs involved are also a factor.

With advancement of technology and better connectivity at high dependability rates, telepresence surgery evolved into telesurgery. Since the robots actually perform the precision surgeries with guidance from a surgeon physically located at some distance (which may be a couple of metres away), the physical distances between the two do not really matter for the surgeon may physically be present in the same room or the room next or even half way across the world.

Networking Connectivity

This is a vitally important consideration since many telemedicine encounters have fallen flat due to this being less than satisfactory. It must be recognised that such connections not only need to conform to a baseline connection speed but the entire processing is data volume-hungry, all of which need access to high-speed Internet connectivity with sufficient data size plans. Such plans are not cheap and the fact that both the clinician and the patient need to have them at either end must be borne in mind before even contemplating offering any type of telemedicine services.

All too often the costing factors in those are incurred in providing the service, while the corresponding costs of receiving them are overlooked. This is a significant mistake for quite often many patients baulk at such services due to the high costs incurred by them in terms of devices (which they have to procure), connectivity (which they have to pay for) and the service charges (which the clinician charges for providing the services). Consequently, it is always a good idea to charge as low as possible for providing the services and recover the costs as goodwill earned or as part of the whole "services rendered" package. *This aspect is discussed in some greater detail in the pricing section in a subsequent chapter.*

Networking connectivity using smartphones can be carried out using data plans from the various service providers serving the area. However, these are usually pricey and should ideally be used only when no nearby Wi-Fi (wireless fidelity) connections are available. Some laptops and all desktops will connect through LAN cables that are plug and play, although the ubiquitous presence of physical cabling running all over the place is usually a source of great annoyance all round.

Wi-Fi access enablement usually involves turning the feature on (readers will do well to note that this feature is power-hungry and will drain the battery faster; so, it should be turned off when not required). Normally the device will "discover" all nearby Wi-Fi access. Public access ones should be avoided like the plague as they are "open" and can easily be "snooped" on. Choose one that is secure. The downside is that it will require a password to be entered to gain access.

There are two other networking methods that are becoming quite popular. One is Bluetooth® and the other near-field communication (NFC)). The problem with these two is that these protocols require the devices to be near each other for effective communication and the problem of battery drainage when not in use but not switched off. Bluetooth devices need to be "paired" before they connect to each other, making them difficult to hack into. However, many devices that use older versions will automatically try to get connected to the one that it was last connected to. Additionally, as soon as another device tries to connect, the previously connected device gets disconnected or "bumped off". All of these are not only annoying but can pose a potential hazard in healthcare monitoring. Consequently, these need to be used with due care. A tentative list of the major types of connectivity is as follows:

1. Wi-Fi
2. Bluetooth

3. NFC
4. ZigBee
5. Modbus
6. Infrared
7. Direct cabling
8. Leased line

A brief description of the various aspects of connectivity related to its architecture with respect to structure (topology) and types is provided below.

Networking Architecture

This is the logical and structural layout of a network. It consists of transmission equipments, software and the various communication protocols (mentioned above) and the infrastructure (wired or wireless) that are used to establish connectivity between components for data transmission.

Networking Topologies

The term "topology" means "arrangement". There are principally five such networking arrangements as follows:

1. Star
2. Bus (or line)
3. Loop (or ring)
4. Tree topology
5. Mesh topology

A sixth type is called hybrid that is basically a mixture of any two or more different types of the other topologies.

> *In the figures depicting the various types of topologies below, all devices like PCs, laptops, printers, handheld devices, servers, etc. have been showed using a common image of a server. This has been done purely for simplification.*

Star Topology

This is a centralised networking architecture where a central node is connected to a number of remote nodes. The remote nodes are not connected to each other but can interconnect through the central node (Fig. 5.1).

Bus (or Line) Topology

In this topology, every device is connected to each other using a single cable (Fig. 5.2).

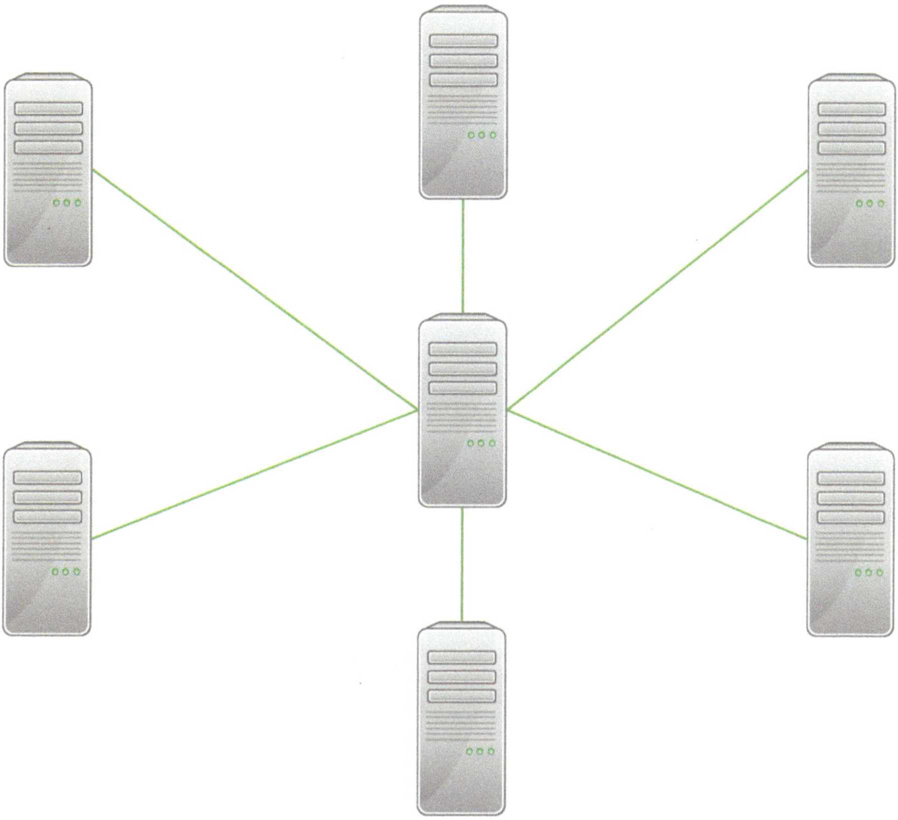

Fig. 5.1 Centralised (hub and spoke) architecture

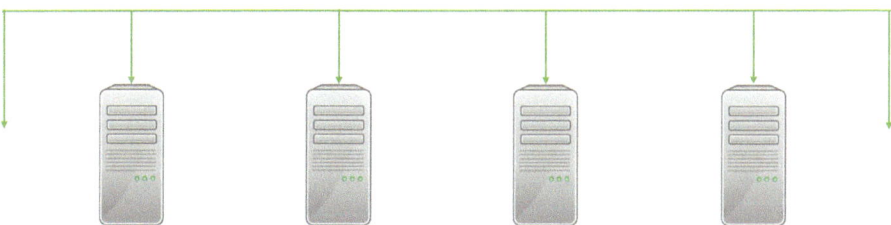

Fig. 5.2 Bus (or line) topology

Loop (or Ring) Topology

In this topology, each device is attached to the other in a ring formation, with the last one connected to the first. It is worth noting that there are exactly two neighbours for each device (Fig. 5.3).

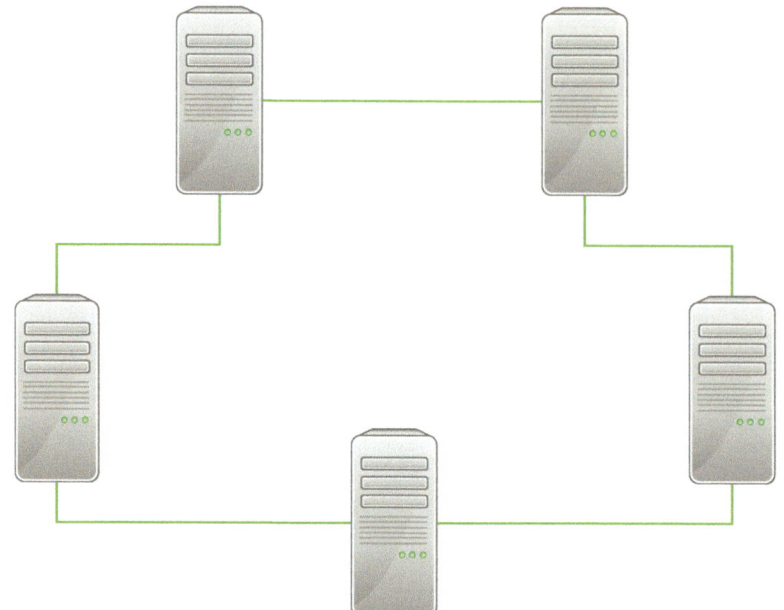

Fig. 5.3 Loop (or ring) topology

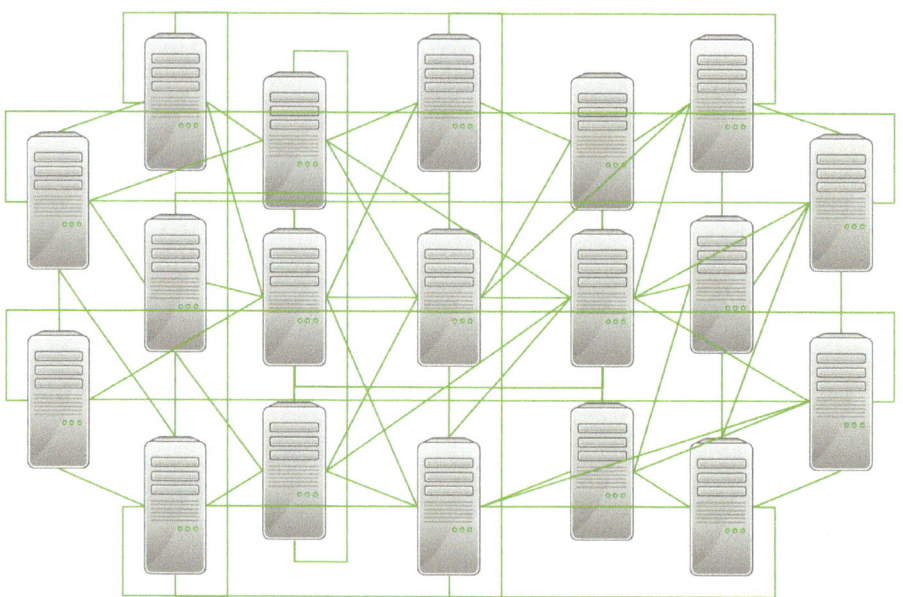

Fig. 5.4 Mesh topology

Mesh Topology

In this topology, the devices use point-to-point connections to connect to other nodes or devices. It is useful to note that all the network nodes are connected to each other. This architecture is typically used by the "network of networks" or the Internet (Fig. 5.4).

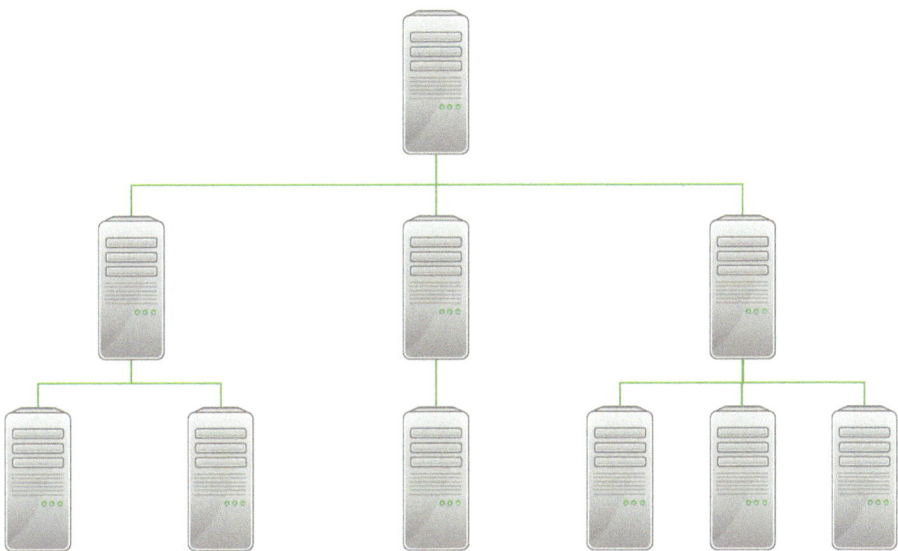

Fig. 5.5 Tree topology

Tree Topology

In this topology, there is a root node and all other nodes are connected to it in a hierarchical manner, and it is therefore also called hierarchical topology. It is necessary that the topology has at least three levels to be considered to form a tree-like topology (Fig. 5.5).

Hybrid Topology

This type of topology is composed of a mixture of two or more topologies. For example, if an organisation uses ring topology in one department and star topology in another, then connecting these two different types of topologies will result in hybrid topology that is composed of ring topology and star topology in this instance.

Network Types

The various types of network are classified according to the geographical areas they cover and named as local area network, metropolitan area network and wide area network.

Local Area Network

A local area network (LAN) connects a group of computers that are in close proximity to each other, like on the same floor or in an office building, within a school complex or just in the apartment or a home. Usually such networks share IT resources and services like electronic files, computer printers, computer games, computer applications, email or very commonly Internet access. They typically are capable of serving many hundreds of connected users. Typically, LAN includes many wires and cables and as well as Wi-Fi (when it gets called WLAN, acronym for wireless local area network). Traditional home networks are typically LANs or more likely WLANs. It is quite possible to have multiple WLANs within one home, like if a "guest" network with distinct access restrictions (user identifiers and pass-words) separated from the "home" network is set up side by side. Hotels typically have such multiple networks meant to serve different purposes. Such separate net-works also help in placing restrictions as appropriate.

Metropolitan Area Network

A metropolitan area network (MAN) interconnects users with computer resources within a single geographic area or region like a postal district or a small town. The term is also applied to interconnections of several local area networks that are located within a common "metropolitan" area. Several such networks in turn may be interconnected to form an efficient wide area network. These types of networks are extremely efficient in terms of reliability and speed and are able to provide fast communication using high-speed data carriers, such as fibre optic cables. Laying such cables proves expensive for LAN but is extremely cost-effective for MANs.

Wide Area Network

A wide area network (WAN) is a communication network that spans a large geo-graphic area such as across cities, states or even countries. They can be "private" connecting parts of a business or more "public" connecting smaller networks together. This type of networking ensures that computers in one location can com-municate with computers in other locations with both ease and efficiency and is implemented with the help of either public transmission systems or private net-works. *Incidentally, the Internet is an example of WAN.*

Typically, local area networks are connected to a wide area network using suit-able intercommunication devices, like a router. The WANs allow the various con-nected users to share access to various applications, services and other centrally located resources. This eliminates the need to have installations of the same applica-tion server, firewall or other resource in multiple locations, which are then shared on-demand instead.

Managed Leased Line Network[2]

This topic deserves a separate section since by using such connections, a number of issues related to reliability and security can be addressed by using such a network. There is a price to be paid for this, but many would find that this is well worth it.

A highly secured, dedicated, communication facility that is available at all times and not shared with anyone else is being increasingly preferred by many business entities. An exclusive leased line provides a dedicated telecommunication path between two fixed points and is capable of carrying voice, data and video. It can be used to connect computers, videoconferencing equipment, telephones and VPN at very high speeds. When the service providers of such leased lines are able to pro-vide end-to-end control and monitor their performance while guaranteeing their uptime, the leased lines are termed as "managed leased lines".

---

[2] electronicsforu.com/technology-trends/managed-leased-line-network.

While there are many applications and services that can be offered using MLLN, like speech, data and international leased circuits, it is the ability to provide private data network that is of particular interest to the healthcare industry. Through such networks, more than one local or long-distance leased circuits can be provided such that data from one leased circuit can automatically be transferred to another for the same subscriber.

The MLLN architecture is a three-tier structure and comprises of network elements such as digital cross connects (DXC), versatile multiplexer (VMUX), network termination units (NTU) and network management system (NMS).

In healthcare, particularly in the context of providing telemedicine services, there is definitely a case to be made for such dedicated and managed leased line circuits that is able to guarantee high quality of service (QoS), efficiency, secured network at desired bandwidth, time-dependent bandwidth provisioning, congestion-free, centralised control and monitoring, lower lead time for new installation and proactive fault maintenance at affordable rates that makes MLLN a boon for all the stakeholders.

Readers are requested to kindly note that MLLN and VPN are two separate beasts. While the former offers reliability in terms of connectivity and bandwidth, the latter provides encryption and authentication over an already available connection. Thus, the need for VPN does not go away simply because one is using a leased line connection.

Any additional information regarding this topic is considered to be out-of-scope for this book. Interested readers are encouraged to refer to the source mentioned or other similar sources.

Virtual Private Network

A VPN is a special type of network that is dynamically constructed on connection using public networks—usually the Internet—to connect to a private network, such as a company's internal network that uses private addresses to identify machines existing within it to communicate with each other. The data exchanged using such networks are quite secure as the networking address required to identify and authenticate the communicating machines to each other is kept private making them extremely protected from hacking.

Issues Related to the Last Mile (Kilometre) Connectivity

The "last mile (or last kilometre) connectivity" is a colloquial phrase (the term "mile" being employed metaphorically) that refers to the final section of a telecommunications network used to deliver telecommunication services to the users. This last (or first, if viewed from the end-user's perspective) mile is typically the speed bottleneck in communication networks as its bandwidth capacity effectively determines the data bandwidth that is actually available to the users.

This is due to the fact that these final mile links happen to be the most numerous and thus represents the most expensive part of the system. It needs to be interfaced with a wide variety of end-user equipment, thereby proving to be the most difficult portion of the entire communication network to upgrade. For example, telephone lines that carry phone calls between switching centres are made of modern optical fibre, but the last mile is typically connected using the century-old technology of phone cables that use twisted pair copper wires. The latter are unable to handle the higher bandwidths that are delivered by the former, thereby leading to consequent bottleneck since the connection speeds follow the principle of lowest common denominator where the lowest speed becomes the effective speed.

To resolve this issue, or at least mitigate it to an optimal extent, service providers often mix the networks like using Wi-Fi to provide the last mile connectivity. Various solutions currently being used include WiMAX and broadband over power lines.

Software

These are actually what makes telemedicine deliver on its full range of promises.

Store and Forward Records

It is always preferable, even if it is not always practicable, to have as much of patient information available during any type of telemedicine session. Since the costs of such consultations are high due to the various operational and connectivity expenses, every second saved results in higher patient satisfaction. Having to hunt around for the correct information is consequently not a very efficient way of conducting such sessions. With the consultation being of an "online" nature, the records too need to be online so that consultant may review and annotate them in real time and make the same being simultaneously available to the patient.

To facilitate this, the need to have "store-and-forward" features is necessary. Using a variety of techniques and technologies to go along with it, the clinician and his patient are able to take pictures including scanned documents like laboratory reports or investigation results, record sounds and videos and record texts before storing them either on some device like the smartphone or tablet or USB stick or in some dedicated storage place like a file server that is preferably located in the Cloud. These may then be exchanged as necessary between them by uploading and downloading or accessing the necessary documents with relative ease and at any location using any suitably connected device 24 × 7.

Mobility Apps

Applications that run on mobility devices like smartphones, tablets, laptops, PDA, etc. are called mobility apps. These apps (short form of applications and generally meant to be used on devices like smartphones and handheld devices) have their own positives and negatives. These are chiefly in terms of installation file sizes (smaller than regular applications), storage capabilities (hardly any) and connectivity with some remote server (most need continuous connection although a few can work without connectivity but still require period reconnections to the Cloud for updating and data synchronisation).

The beauty of these apps is in their graphics (very rich), ease of use (users only need to use their fingers—hand gestures—to accomplish most tasks) and ability to empower users to perform actions with minimum of effort as they are able to utilise the various functionalities offered by the mobility devices like responsive screens, motion sensors, gyroscopes, GPS, camera, microphone, speaker, etc.

Health Apps

From a health point of view, many health apps are already available that are able to track and provide health-related tips based on the various activities like steps walked, floors climbed, distance walked, calories ingested, etc. of the user. These apps are able to help users follow a healthy lifestyle and alert them for any deviations (from preset goals) so that they can take the necessary corrective measures and lead a healthy life.

Homecare Apps

These mobility apps are geared especially for providing homecare. Such apps are able to alert the user throughout the day by waking them up to their favourite tune or radio station, prompt them regarding any tests they need to take (like checking fasting blood glucose level) and medications to take and track calories ingested (the user can take the picture and fill in some additional details of what all they are eating and the app can inform the amount of calories it contains), time to have a meal, time to go for a walk, time to go to sleep, etc.

All such apps can prove to be real life-savers as they can track the movement, or lack thereof, of the user. Should someone have a fainting spell or suddenly stop moving (tracked using GPS and motion sensors), the remotely located carer using predictive analytics, like signal processing, can instantaneously be alerted and immediate action initiated like making a phone call to find out whether the person being monitored is alright or even send across a fully staffed ambulance with all necessary life-saving equipment to save the patient from any major health-related life event.

There is one big downside to this. After a while it can become somewhat irritating as the app almost becomes a *de facto* "big nanny" that many would find to be rather bothersome.

Remote Monitoring Solutions

When monitoring, either bedside or remote, a single monitoring solution includes a dashboard to provide all information integrated and at a glance preferably with some inbuilt intelligence to raise warning signals and alerts based on preset criteria that the clinician may take cognisance of and intervene, proactively in many cases, to ensure delivery of optimal care. Readers will note that a nursing station is actually a remote location, and all that can be displayed and monitored from a conveniently located nursing station can also be displayed and monitored from any other location, provided connectivity between the connected locations exist.

Messaging Apps

These have become so ubiquitous that it is almost impossible to meet someone who has not used one in the recent past or is not an active regular user. If someone has a smartphone, which almost everyone appears to have one these days, then it is wise to presume that that person is using some messaging app of some sort.

With many such messenger apps providing end-to-end encryption making data exchange between them extremely secure, they are increasingly being used for exchanging health-related information, and many clinicians and patients alike are using these as their preferred mode of exchanging results, reports, feedback, advice, etc. Taking advantage of the various features of mobility devices like the ability to take pictures (still and motion), capture sounds, read bar/QR codes, etc., video chatting, telepresence, scanning and displaying documents (like reports, notes, etc.), through its various functionalities the messaging applications have brought the ability to conduct decent telepresence interaction and easy exchange of information of any kind to the users. Virtual reality (VR) can help either parties (patient or provider) to get a "feel" that they are right next to each other, and when coupled with haptics, it is possible to even do "virtual touching". To use these for telemedicine purposes is not only pretty straightforward but not using them is most likely a great disservice to the patient.

One should however exercise due caution when using these applications especially in healthcare settings. As long as there is faith and trust, anything goes. However, in cases of distrust and when litigations can and do happen for any reason, the courts of law and professional councils with power of oversight and ability to punish for breaches of law and ethics are bound to take an extremely dim view of the seemingly blatant disregard of matters related to privacy, secrecy and confidentiality.

The bottom line is that clinicians must take extreme care and display great sensitivity when using these apps for providing care. *This aspect is discussed in more details in the chapter dealing with the various legal aspects.*

Connected Health

This is a newly introduced sociotechnical model that uses telemedicine technology to remotely provide various healthcare services remotely. Its aim is to maximise healthcare resources and provide increased flexible opportunities for patients to engage with their clinicians and better manage their care themselves. This model encompasses terms such as digital health, eHealth, mHealth, telehealth, telehomecare, remote care and active assisted living (AAL).

A variety of devices, instruments and equipments located in homes and clinics are connected to backend databases via devices located at the site that act as some localised central hub for data aggregation. These devices, which act as "aggregation devices" of sorts, are themselves usually dedicated device gateways, home routers, smartphones and even PCs.[3] Incidentally, the networking type thus formed is often referred to as a personal area network (PAN).

Commonly accepted network interface standards like Wi-Fi, Bluetooth®, NFC, ZigBee, etc. are employed to interconnect the various health devices and the aggregation device. Similarly, the interface between the aggregation device and the patient medical records is governed by regulations that mandate using certain approved standards and certifications. These include Personal Connected Health Alliance Profiles and the ISO/IEEE 11703-20601 Optimized Exchange protocols.

Unfortunately, many device manufacturers and vendors do not support these standards in their products. This leads to an unhelpful state of affairs as significant interoperability issues on a continued basis, and consequent increased system integration costs hamper their increased adoption and widespread use overall, especially within the telemedicine paradigm.

Internet of Things[4]

The Internet of things (stylised Internet of Things or IoT) is the inter-networking of "things" represented by physical devices, vehicles (also referred to as "connected devices" and "smart devices"), buildings and other items—embedded with electronics, software, sensors, actuators and network connectivity that enable these objects to collect and exchange data. Typically, IoT is expected to offer advanced connectivity of devices, systems and services that goes beyond machine-to-machine (M2M) communications and covers a variety of protocols, domains and applications.

As of 2016, the vision of the Internet of things has evolved largely due to a convergence of multiple technologies, including ubiquitous wireless communication, real-time analytics, machine learning, commodity sensors and embedded systems. This means that the traditional fields of embedded systems, wireless sensor networks, control systems, automation (including home and building automation) and others all contribute to enabling the Internet of things.

Internet of Healthcare Things
When the "things" mentioned above relate to healthcare, the result is an Internet of healthcare things (IoHT). The various healthcare "things" could be wearables, apps, monitors, etc., that are connected to other "things" or a central system that performs

---

[3] Personal computer.

[4] Harnessing big data analytics to deliver optimal care. Dr. SB Bhattacharyya. Asian Hospital and Health Management, April 2017 (www.asianhhm.com/information-technology/harnessing-big-data-analytics-deliver-optimal-care).

storage, analysis and monitoring via aggregation devices, mentioned above, that are located at the patient's site.

Currently, many of the "wearables" in the shape of a wristband or smartwatch are being used by many as personal health monitoring devices. These too qualify as "healthcare things", and through their ability to connect to a smartphone or a similar mobility device that acts as aggregation devices, the captured data is transmitting through a health monitoring server located (most likely) in the Cloud that runs machine learning algorithms to help the wearers maintain a healthy lifestyle especially from a wellness and preventive care perspective.

Underlying Privacy and Information Dependability Aspects

These are major concerns in telemedicine, particularly in telemonitoring and remote care. In order to be workable within the clinical care paradigm, the remote patient monitoring systems need to ensure that both the patient privacy and information quality of the data that are generated by the biosensors and monitors are respected and maintained on a continued basis. There are many ways in which data can be lost or become undependable or get exposed to hacking. Some very plausible examples are the monitors or sensors being incorrectly applied, misplacing or losing the device itself (being expensive some may be stolen), or become compromised as the data travels through multiple devices and communication networks, many of which are wireless, before being made available for analysis (by a machine and/or care providers).

As can be easily comprehended, vulnerabilities such as these are totally unacceptable in any healthcare setting, just telemedicine. Faulty data belonging to the wrong patient adds to totally avoidable morbidity and mortality as well as makes healthcare professionals to become generally distrustful of not only the data but also in the technology itself. The patients too may refuse to use such devices if they are unable to trust that their privacy is not guaranteed and confidential information may be exposed without them even being aware of such breaches. It is human to err. Even with proper training, people who need to use them do make even silly mistakes quite commonly.[5]

However, using smartphones and other similar handheld devices like tablets and PDAs for healthcare comes with challenges of their own. Each sensor needs to use different software to make them run making them vulnerable to their exploitation of their design flaws. The devices themselves need to use a variety of connectivity mechanisms to function properly. All of these need to be carefully factored in when developing applications that make them to work in concert effectively, something that healthcare almost routinely requires.

---

[5] Secure Remote Health Monitoring with Unreliable Mobile Devices; Minho Shin; Myongji University, Yongin, Gyeonggi-do 449–728, Republic of Korea; Hindawi Publishing Corporation, Journal of Biomedicine and Biotechnology, Volume 2012, Article ID 546021.

For example, the remote monitoring system may be interacting with the patient using telepresence while simultaneously checking his weight, BP, pulse rate, temperature and partial pressure of oxygen saturation. To add to this, it should be verifiable that the data being streamed through to the remote care monitoring system does belong to the same person, has a date and time stamp and is not garbled.

One way of addressing the security concerns would be to transmit the data through a password-protected Wi-Fi router and encrypt them using full AES-128 or AES-196 or even AES-256 encryption algorithms before transmission. The remotely located clinicians may subsequently access it by logging in to a web portal[6] that uses role-based access control to address the underlying privacy, confidentiality and secrecy concerns.

Data Vulnerability

This is a big issue for all electronic media irrespective of whether it is healthcare related or not. People are apprehensive and all the ghastly stories that get reported almost on a daily basis make this a very justifiable emotion.

It is generally accepted that "data is as secure as at its weakest point". Gaining unauthorised access to or hacking into any system is performed by exploiting the weakest point in the system. Most of the time, this is due to the use of weak passwords that makes gaining access by anyone, either self or friend or foe, literally a child's play. Routers are also another weak point with most routers having a pretty standard default access credentials in terms of user identifier and password (*unique id/password* = *admin/password*) and web address URL. While all routers have features that can make accessing the administrator's panel very secure, unless done by those who know how to properly set it up, it can lead to disaster and untold misery. Hence, it is definitely the money well spent to hire a professional and pay him good money to do it if one does not know how to do it himself.

All users need to log in to the system to gain access and use its various functionalities. For this, a unique identifier and an associated password are required to uniquely identify and authenticate the person logging in. This password is really the key since it is only supposed to be known to the user and no other human. Ideally, no one else should be able to read it as it is stored in an encrypted form in the system that only it can comprehend. Systems usually mask the entered characters (including text, numbers and special characters) with asterisks ("*"), to prevent even the user from seeing it lest someone else looks over their shoulders without their knowledge and is able to learn it. Should the user forget it, he needs to reset it and use a new one.

While this is all very well, it must be recognised that this process is not "idiot proof"—if the user himself chooses to compromise by using a very weak password that anyone else can easily guess, like using as their preferred password the word

---

[6] Secured Smart Healthcare Monitoring System Based on IoT; Bhoomika. B. K, Dr. K N Muralidhara; PES college of Engineering, Mandya; (www.ijritcc.org/download/1438757194.pdf).

"password" itself or "abc123" or their name or date of birth, etc, and, worse, if the user for reasons of his own chooses to tell someone else his password. Once anyone is able to learn the password by means foul or fair, hacking into the system is but a child's play.

Without going into too much details, passphrases (for which the readers are encouraged to refer to the registration methodology advocated in a later chapter), personal identification number (PIN) and even biometrics like fingerprint, thumb print, palm scan, retinal scan, iris scan, etc., have been made use of. Adoption of such authentication techniques does certainly make the system more difficult, if not impossible, to break in.

A good yet simple process would be to periodically change passwords (or use passphrases composed of words picked at random that may or may not have any spaces in between), for example, every 21–30 days,[7] and never reuse any previously used password/passphrase or at least not the last three or five.

One must always be cautious of exchanging information with unknown persons. Any person contacting others using a compromised machine can also compromise the machine belonging to the contacted person. This can happen even without the person contacting being completely unaware of the fact that he is using a compromised machine.

It must always however be borne in mind that all these measures (password/passphrase management, using PIN and/or biometrics, end-to-end encryption, etc.) help minimise risks but not totally eliminate them.

Another extremely important thing to remember is that all systems need to be kept periodically updated, particularly the operating systems, without any exceptions. Firewalls and anti-virus software help in keeping machines safe. Prudence and prior knowledge regarding phishing—a good tip to adopt wholeheartedly—is never to click on any links in emails even if they look to have sent by someone whom one knows.

Legal versions of paid software are usually safe, but illegal versions and free software from unknown sources are pretty vulnerable. In the modern day and age, ignorance is not bliss and foolhardy instead for one must be extremely careful in ensuring the genuineness of nearly everything.

Telemedicine Services Architecture

These draw inspiration from the networking topologies mentioned above. The difference is that it depicts the way the various telemedicine centres, from where services may be offered, are interconnected to facilitate sharing of resources and covering a wider area (of both service area and range of services). It substitutes the computer devices with telemedicine centres and services.

---

[7] To force password change every day is an overkill and one every 3 months too lax; the mentioned range is just about okay.

Hub and Spoke

Similar to Star Topology

Within the telemedicine services paradigm, this type of topology is considered to be the most efficient as one central location can simultaneously be connected to a number of remote ones. It is not necessary that all can be active simultaneously and can be connected one after another with minimum disruptions. This makes good sense in teleconsultations as only one encounter can take place between a patient and clinician at any one given point in time.

Usually, the clinician is placed at the central node and the patients the remote ones at the end of the "spokes". This may however be reversed if a single patient is being cared for by a number of clinicians like in critical care where a patient is cared for by a consultant, an intensivist, several nurses, paramedics, nutritionist, physiotherapist, etc.

Federated

Similar to Hybrid Topology

In this architecture several centralised architectures are interconnected to each other where one acts like the hub and the others as spokes. Within the telemedicine services paradigm, this type of topology can be used when several teleconsultation centres decide to collaborate with each other while providing telemedicine services. One of the networks can connect to another thereby sharing resources amongst themselves.

For example, using such a networking structure, a single nutritionist will be able to provide teleconsultations to several more persons without having to be a part of several teleconsultation facilities if the facilities participate in a federated manner and provide the opportunity for such a collaboration to take place (Fig. 5.6).

Distributed

Similar to Mesh Topology

Within the telemedicine services paradigm, this is the networking topology of choice for providing telemonitoring and remote care services. If the interconnected servers are assumed to be themselves connected to various devices like videoconferencing, EHR systems, patient monitors, medical devices, wearables, etc., that are either attached to or gathering data from persons with the various health portals and handheld devices like smartphones, tablets or laptops acting as display units, etc., then it is not difficult to visualise how all of them will be able to collaborate to collect the required data from and provide the latest information to the various stakeholders in real time without any delay.

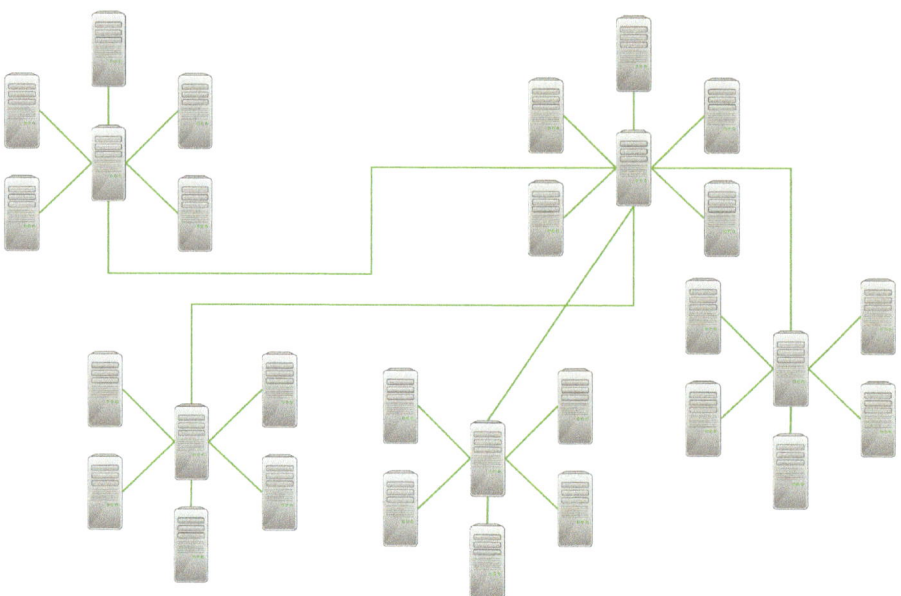

Fig. 5.6 Federated architecture

Overview and General Principles

6

Abstract

This chapter deals with the general principles that have been followed in the actual DIY Guide parts. While those aspects that are specific to a particular service type like teleconsultation or telemonitoring or remote care are dealt with dedicated chapters of their own, the aspects that are common to all of them are discussed in this chapter.

Overview

If any patient is being "seen" for the very first time, it is advisable to examine the patient in person and not remotely. Should a patient be an "old" patient whom one has not only examined before but is now seeking advice for what can essentially be classified as a "follow-up" encounter or is looking for a review of an ongoing problem that merits no physical examination, then teleconsultation may be considered as an alternative to an in-person visit.

At the end of the day, all things considered, it is the clinician's call to decide whether the patient needs to be physically present in front of him or will teleconsultation suffice.

For telemonitoring or telereferral or remote care situations, telemedicine works quite well as here only a review is carried out and advice provided either to someone physically present with the patient in the form of a care provider or carer to carry out (telemonitoring or telereferral) or the patient himself (remote care).

It needs to be mentioned here that both telesurgery and tele-CME are valid types of application of telemedicine technology. However, the aim of this book is to guide single clinicians who wish to use telemedicine to help deliver better care to their patients and thereby increase patient satisfaction while reducing their stress, hopefully. Hence, only teleconsultation, telemonitoring and remote care have been dealt with, while telesurgery and tele-CME have not.

© Springer Nature Singapore Pte Ltd. 2017
S.B. Bhattacharyya, *A DIY Guide to Telemedicine for Clinicians*,
DOI 10.1007/978-981-10-5305-4_6

Components

Any good messaging application that supports video-, audio- and text-based chats permits exchanging files of any type—although the use of a Cloud-based file storage system preferably with facilities for private access occasionally works better—plus an EHR system that is preferably Cloud based.

The ideal solution will perhaps be some smartphone- or tablet-based open-source app that is a composite of video and audio chat, text messaging and secure and private file exchange system integrated with an EHR system. However, as of early 2017, such an application does not exist. So, clinicians would need to make do with ones that can be considered to be good substitutes, albeit through a careful and creative use of several apps in combination it is quite possible to get the same tasks done without much ado.

IoT or IoHT (Internet of Things or Internet of Healthcare Things) would be something that is bound to be heard of more in the near future. Once the appropriate solutions are available to the end users, it would ideally involve no more than logging in to an application on a device and attaching the various "healthcare things" to it. The rest of the activities including coordination will be handled deep in the background, about which the end user will largely be completely unware of while using the system.

Setting It Up

Usually the following will need to be used:

1. A messaging app that permits, preferably in an encrypted manner to make
   (a) Video calls
   (b) Audio calls
   (c) Text messaging
2. A Cloud-based file sharing application that permits private file sharing on a one-to-one basis
3. A Cloud-based EHR system where the patient and the clinician are both registered (a dedicated stand-alone system will also do, although a "true" EHR may not be available in such instances)
4. A high-speed Internet connection (2 mbps+ Internet connection with sufficient bandwidth of 2 GB+ per month for patient and 20 GB+ per month for clinician provided the clinician does not need to review high-grade DICOM image files, i.e. any CT, MRI or PET scans)

It is assumed that a smart device, in the form of a smartphone or tablet or wearable, or a PC in the form of laptop or a desktop is available at both ends – the patient and the provider. It is also assumed that the device or computer is attached to the Internet with a suitable data and net connectivity plan. Other than the about-to-be or already obsolete desktop PC, most of the other devices come equipped with high-quality video and audio facilities in terms of camera, microphone, screen display and audio equipment in terms of speakers and microphones by default that may be made good use of for most if not all face-to-face interactions.

The proclivity to use the same messaging app that is being used for telemedicine for purposes other than that by the clinicians should be strongly resisted to ensure that a certain degree of professionalism is maintained and the messages do not get mixed up, thereby compromising the patient's privacy and confidentiality.

Since this book is not meant for patients, aspects dealing with how they should be setting up and using the various components are not dealt here. Nevertheless, it should be mentioned here that they will need to use the same messaging system that their clinicians are using for obvious reasons.

Registering

This activity should ideally need to be done only once but is the most important step to start using any service. Usually during the process, one must register oneself by providing certain personal details and choosing an appropriate username and a strong password or better still a passphrase.

Some dos and don'ts related to registration and use of passwords are as follows:

1. Do use an easy-to-remember username.
2. Do supply the minimum required information.
3. Do not use any tacky username.
4. Do use strong passwords with a combination of uppercase, lowercase, special characters and numbers; and the total length of the passwords should be of lengths not less than eight characters.
5. Do use passphrase wherever possible using a combination of unrelated and randomly chosen words, preferably not less than four (4), and separated by a blank space or not—apparently the rather difficult to type but easy to pronounce passphrase "ilovefreshsashimitunawithalittlesoyandwasabi" (*without spaces, with spaces it is "I love fresh sashimi tuna with a little soy and wasabi"*) will require 10,000+ centuries to break by brute-force method using an average home computer as currently (early 2017) available.[1]
6. Do not post the chosen password or passphrase anywhere (email, social media, messaging apps, etc.) or share it with anyone.

Once the registration process is successful, the username of the clinician needs to be shared with the patients so that they may add them to their application to start interacting. Alternatively, it is useful to ask the patients to share their username so that the clinician can add them to his list of contacts. A separate contact group of patients is useful to maintain separate professional contacts from personal ones.

---

[1] https://password.kaspersky.com/.

Running It

An unwritten but a very important rule to bear in mind is "when in doubt, ask the patient to come and visit the clinician for a physical encounter in person".

Telemedicine Session

For those clinicians who have their usual clinic timings, it is preferable to have specific timings dedicated exclusively for conducting telemedicine sessions. Else, things tend to become somewhat complicated with either the patient in person or the patient in virtual feeling neglected due to their time (and consequently space) being constantly and irritatingly intruded upon.

Initiating
At the scheduled time (or unscheduled one), the "call" can be initiated by either the patient or the clinician as has (preferably) been decided before. This is done by clicking the appropriate menu item or button to initiate a telepresence session or audio chat. For text messaging, the user starts typing their messages immediately after selecting the addressee.

One should always start with a friendly greeting. Then the conversation should proceed as if it were a face-to-face encounter. No distractions of any kind, like talking to someone else or taking a call or leaving the seat (unless for a "comfort break"), should be permitted. The person at the other end will not be appreciative of such gestures as these tend to show a certain degree of disrespect and undervaluation of the time and effort being put in. This is true for both the patient and the clinician alike, the latter especially so.

Connecting
Usually the connection is automatic and performed by the messaging system. Occasionally, the connectivity can be less than optimal leading to distorted video images, garbled audio and delayed delivery of text messages. In such circumstances, it would be better to end the session and reinitiate it either immediately or as soon as possible. For handheld devices using GPRS/GSM/CDMA, physically moving to a location where better connectivity is present generally helps. Once a good connectivity has been achieved, it is generally advisable for either party not to move around too much.

Establishing connection is a tricky business. Largely dependent on the type of device and the way they connect, it could mean anything from syncing with another device that acts as an aggregating device (data collection hub) on a one-to-one basis to cabling them to each other directly. All monitors/sensors will come with their own set of instructions for use and interconnection. These need to be consulted as often as required. Occasionally, expert help is required. Whenever any device is bought, it is necessary to ensure that installation support, preferably by an expert, is provided along with.

The first thing that one must do once the connection has been established and friendly greetings exchanged is to ensure that the correct consent is taken. The patient should be apprised of his rights and privileges and his agreement to continuing with the session needs to be taken before proceeding. Needless to state, if the consent is not forthcoming to the satisfaction of both the patient and the clinician, the session should immediately be terminated, with politeness but firmness.

Video Chat

Also Telepresence Sessions

Bright lighting always helps. Although most video cameras are able to display images even at 0 lux (zero luminosity or no light), it is better assumed that their image-intensification abilities will not be enough to surmount all shortcomings. The lacunas they produce make reliance on the generated images risky, especially in a clinical context as the remote-located clinician will have to rely on his acumen to get the "right" picture.

Audio Chat

Audio chats without a concomitant video are a little tricky. Most of these would be over a phone call. As has been mentioned before, communication consists of visual and aural components of which the former is significantly larger than the latter. Once the visual component is eliminated from the equation, the major component of the messaging paradigm is actually lost, and the listener is forced to "fill in" the gaps mentally. Occasionally, this "filling in" occurs by judging the intonations and inflections of the aural component, making the process inherently imperfect. This results in "lost in translation" to varying degrees that might prove to be particularly problematic in a "clinical" context.

Text Messaging

A frequently used and very convenient way of exchanging information, text messaging has come a long way since being constrained by the character limitations and high costs of exchanging them imposed by SMS service providers. What it loses through the absence of both the visual and the aural components in their entirety, it gains in clarity provided by the written testament of the information. In combination with audio-video messaging, the level of clarity gained is probably at its highest. One must be mindful of spelling errors, faulty grammar and poor language skills, not forgetting the irritation caused by the automatic spellchecks that arbitrarily autocorrect words and manage to produce amusing and often disastrous instances of what can only mildly be referred to as "word salad". Consequently, one must be mindful of the fact that the potential to add to both morbidity and mortality is too great to ignore.

Netiquette

Saying "hello", "please" and "thank you" in any language is always a good thing. So, it is both important to be polite and courteous at all times. One will do well to remember that all telemedicine sessions requires professionalism to be continuously displayed.

Using the following is better avoided at all times:

1. Capital letters—they denote shouting in text messaging and emails.
2. Too many emojis—they are distracting.
3. Acronyms—the other party may not understand them clearly.
4. Difficult-to-understand language.
5. Harsh, belittling or derogatory words.
6. Too long text messages—short ones are easier to read and comprehend.

File Sharing

There are two widely used methods for this.

1. Directly transferring the file using the messaging service—the advantage is that the exchange is one to one and hence cannot easily be hacked into; the disadvantage is that depending upon the connection speed, large files are difficult to exchange (for speeds, the lowest speed at any end prevails; hence, if the speed is 256 kbps at one end and 16 mbps at the other, the files will get exchanged at 256 kbps speeds!).
2. Using a dedicated file sharing application located in the Cloud where a file can be uploaded for eventual download by parties to whom access has been granted is very helpful for telemedicine—the advantage is that not only can larger files be uploaded and downloaded outside of the telemedicine session, it can be done asynchronously where the user can perform this activity (upload or download) at a time convenient to him; the disadvantage is that proper access has to be granted to the receiving (downloading-end) party by the sending (uploading-end) party beforehand and if the access is made "public", then anyone may download the file without anyone else being any the wiser, which impacts privacy and confidentiality negatively.

Exchanging Files

Patience is of the essence here. Occasionally the connectivity at one end will not match the other, and so either party may get frustrated when exchanging large files. Fortunately, in medicine, mostly images of CT, MRI or PET scans and HD pictomicrographs tend to be large, while X-rays and USG usually do not. Scanned documents too can be of large sizes, although not the printed ones like prescriptions, investigation results and reports and discharge summaries.

Upload speeds are typically much slower than download speeds (usually ¼). So uploading a file will take time, while downloading the same file will be faster. Data volumes are different from data speeds. So, a 1 GB plan will allow only 1 GB worth of data to be uploaded and/or downloaded for the duration of the plan. So the applicable formula is

$$\text{Data volume} = \text{Total downloaded file size} + \text{Total uploaded file size}$$

Viewing/Playing Files

This depends on the type of file. An indicative table is provided below for quick reference (Table 6.1).

Table 6.1 Handling specific file types

File type	Viewing/rendering method
Text	Web browser/application interface
PDF	PDF viewer (web browser and other interface plug-ins available)
JPEG, TIFF	Image browser/viewer (suitable plug-ins available)
DICOM	DICOM image viewer/monitor
Video file format (e.g. FLV, AVI, WMV, MP4, MPEG, etc.)	Video player capable of playing the particular file format (suitable plug-ins available)
Audio file format (e.g. MP3, WAV, WMA, AIFF, PCM, OGG, etc.)	Audio file player capable of playing the particular file format (suitable plug-ins available)

Ending the Session

The session should be ended with politeness. Once the pleasantries have been exchanged, either party can end the session by choosing the appropriate menu item or clicking the button meant for the purpose. It is usually labelled as "end call" or something similar for video and audio chat. For text it usually is "end session".

Telemonitoring and Remote Care

Here the "context of focus" is the various biosensors and monitors like blood glucometer, pulse oximeters, weighing machines, cardiac pacemakers, etc., and smartphone sensors like accelerometers, GPS, compass, etc., that are connected to the patient for capturing all sorts of health-related data.

Although many devices generate alerts whenever any pre-set limits, both upper and lower, are exceeded, not all have this feature. For that, appropriate application software are required to make "sense" out of the captured data. Acting on the alerts is yet another aspect that, although may be automated, is better handled with at least a certain degree of oversight by trained personnel.

Reviewing

Including offline reviewing

It is necessary to have the "right" kind of application that will allow efficient reviews to occur smoothly. The wave forms, images and sounds can be rendered "as is" to the reviewer. Numerical data can not only be rendered "as is" but also graphically displayed using a variety of graph types.

A word of caution is merited here. Graph types are many. What will work best for whom is highly subjective being more of a matter of individual choice. It is easy to get swayed by the wide range of choices that one has and mess things up a bit. Though the propensity is strong, one must always be conscious of avoiding the omnipresent pitfall called "analysis paralysis" that renders the user incapable of making the "right" set of choices at the "right" time.

It is best to allocate a separate time exclusively for this activity, free from any distractions like attending on or consulting with a patient including conducting a telemedicine session.

Interpreting Device Readings

The readings may be classified broadly into the following three categories:

1. Normal—the reading represents that the data is within normal limits specified for the item that it represents.
2. Abnormal—the reading represents some abnormality due to the patient's physiological state and needs some type of intervention by his clinician
3. Iatrogenic error—the reading represents some abnormality that is not due to the patient's physiological state but due to faults in the devices that may necessitate its re-calibration or even replacement when such errors creep up repeatedly.

Using machine learning techniques like signal processing, logistic regression, K-means clustering and pattern matching can help figure out the veracity of the readings. This may result in certain device readings being totally ignored as being false or triggering rule-based algorithms or alerts or warnings to initiate any follow-on action.

Determining Charges

Costing

Items

1. Device—since this is used for a variety of purposes that include telemedicine, the costs incurred should be amortised elsewhere and not considered exclusive to telemedicine.
2. Video camera.
3. Audio system.
4. Telepresence or video chat/audio chat/text chat/messaging application—generally opt for free; there are plenty of such available; also note that the patient at the other end also needs to have the same application, so a free application is always the first choice.
5. File sharing option—this should ideally belong to the patient who allows access to his doctor, so in effect it's free for the latter.
6. File viewer applications—almost all are free; although sophisticated but expensive DICOM viewers exist, these are mostly of use to the radio-diagnostic professionals and not for routine telemedicine sessions.

7. EHR system depends on the functionalities provided with the better and more useful ones usually requiring some payment in the form of pay per use or subscription or outright purchase.
8. Remote patient monitoring system can end up being the most expensive piece of equipment, particularly if it incorporates machine learning techniques to provide automated alerts and warnings for both the clinician and patients alike that act as inputs for subsequent activity (this is discussed in some detail in a later chapter).
9. Data connection costs depend on the leased line fees or Internet service provider and the data plan opted for and are most likely to be the third most expensive piece of equipment after EHR system and health monitoring devices and also a recurring cost as the service-cum-data plan is usually billed on a monthly basis although the leased lines incur a one-time fixed-cost and an annual subscription fee.
10. Electricity costs—for all health monitoring devices as well as other non-health-related equipment like cameras, display screens, microphones, speakers, lights, furniture, air conditioning, etc.
11. Establishment and infrastructure costs—may be one time to build and recurring for maintenance or recurring rental fees.

Pricing

The readers are requested to refer to the section on pricing telemedicine services in a later chapter of this book for discussion about pricing in detail. Needless to say, this issue can make or break any telemedicine service offering. Charge too little and soon enough find oneself being out of pocket or being saddled with an unviable business. Charge too much and find no takers for the services on offer, no matter how practical they are. Consequently, this needs careful consideration with great sensitivity.

Zero Pricing
The costs are expected to be recovered indirectly through increased revenues due to goodwill and efficiency of care delivery services.

Premium Pricing
Aka markup pricing
   This translates into having a certain markup percentage added to the cost of goods sold, i.e.

$$\text{Price} = \text{Cost of good sold} \times \text{Markup\%}.$$

At Cost Pricing
This translates into not-for-profit or at no-profit-no-loss basis, i.e.

$$\text{Price} = \text{Cost of goods sold}.$$

Estimating I & E Financials

Costs to the patient will include device costs, networking connection costs, power consumption costs, periodic subscription fee for receiving the services and/or clinician visits and consultation costs, etc. These are not considered when calculating for telemedicine services as these are not incurred by the service provider.

Costs to the clinician will include monitoring servers (discussed in a later section), connectivity costs, power consumption costs, establishment costs (the monitoring room will incur a certain cost, like rental, maintenance, etc.), personnel costs (those who will be responsible for the administration of the monitoring system), etc.

Notable Points

1. As in any clinical care setting, the clinician is legally liable for all telemedicine sessions; hence, if at any time the clinician feels that the patient needs to be examined in person, he should insist only on it.
2. Informed patient consent must be taken to cover all locally applicable legal aspects and archive it before doing anything else; notes of all activity should be kept for medico-legal purposes—hence, the need of an EHR/EMR system cannot be overstated as it can demonstrate to everyone's satisfaction the details about a case, what all had been done and what all had not been done with justifications for the decisions taken.
3. Privacy issues must be carefully considered and every piece of information treated as being sacrosanct that is never to be disclosed without explicit permission.
4. When in doubt, one must always check and recheck facts till one is absolutely certain—this is very important in telemedicine as some bits and pieces of information may be missed.
5. At all times, one must factor in the probability that many data may be "lost in transmission" as can happen in the course of any phone call.
6. One must always have a standard operating plan to handle disaster situations like erratic/loss of/no connectivity.

Teleconsultation

7

Abstract

This chapter provides the details as to how teleconsultation services may be offered to patients. The methodology required and steps for setting the services up, running it and performing maintenance of the various equipments and instruments involved are all discussed.

Overview

Teleconsultations are usually conducted only with prior appointment and require the use of high-quality audio-visual equipment in specially designated rooms. It is conducted in a formal setting, and there are at least two ends—the patient's end and clinician's end (the clinician's end can be his consultation chambers).

Other care providers may simultaneously be present in separate locations or at the patient's and/or the clinician's end, either individually or in a group, to conduct a comprehensive review and help in care planning in a collaborative manner within a single teleconsultation session.

A number of equipments like USG scanners capable of performing echocardiograms, vital monitors, ECG machines, digital stethoscopes, etc., may be required at the patient's end where the digital outputs are telemetered through to the clinician's end and rendered over there using display screens, speakers, software solutions, etc., as required.

These sessions must be considered as referral session for all intents and purposes. Consequently, it is imperative that an EHR system be available that can access and display the past EMRs of the patient being reviewed. Without this teleconsultations remain incomplete, leaving the patient short changed. This is neither fair nor wise since any subsequent legal challenges regarding the care or advice delivered will put the clinician on a weaker footing as the fact that "due care" has

© Springer Nature Singapore Pte Ltd. 2017
S.B. Bhattacharyya, *A DIY Guide to Telemedicine for Clinicians*,
DOI 10.1007/978-981-10-5305-4_7

been exercised at all times cannot be proven for lack of sufficient exculpatory evidence to support one's contention.

Teleconsultation is basically telepresence for a special situation. Connectivity thus is a very important issue. The best is a managed leased line network (MLLN) that provides point-to-point connections. Dedicated satellite links work well as the next-best alternative and are the communication links of choice where such end-to-end leased lines cannot be placed. Unfortunately, getting a dedicated satellite transponder or even booking it for a certain time each day is prohibitively expensive unless some subsidy in the form of fee waiver or reduced rates is available. Over the years, ADSL connections have become the medium of choice for most Internet service providers worldwide to provide Internet services to homes and are available for quite high speeds at very affordable costs.

There are both free and open source software (FOSS) as well as commercial telepresence applications available. These use the global Internet Protocol (IP) network and unified communications to deliver an immersive, same-room conferencing experience that is far more powerful and flexible than traditional videoconferencing systems and can be used to provide teleconsultations at relatively low costs.[1]

The connectivity between all the ends too needs to be established and tested out beforehand. Its failure to function optimally during any telemedicine session, let alone teleconsultation, is totally unacceptable.

Methodology

The following are the essential steps. Usually this will be almost identical to any outpatient in-person consultation process.

1. Make an appointment.
   (a) Both the clinician and the patient need to be available for teleconsultation on the date and time as per schedule.
   (b) The initial allotted time slot can be kept at 15 minutes that can be extended by further intervals of 15 minutes for as many number of times as deemed necessary.
   (c) If the consultation is over before the scheduled time, the next appointment can be taken up provided the patient next in the time slot is available. One must ensure that patients are not "passed over" in preference of someone else or that the patient queue is not broken unless there is an overwhelming reason like in an emergency situation when the patients who were not attended to in their usual appointment schedule receive priority appointment in subsequent scheduling—the patient is more than likely to be mightily aggrieved if they are not attended to at their appointed hour, and repeated "bouncing" them off schedule will make them complain about "deficiency of service" or consult someone else.

---

[1] https://en.wikipedia.org/wiki/Telepresence.

(d) One must not forget to make sure that the scheduled maintenance periods are catered to by blocking appropriate time slots for them.

(e) Should an appointment need to be cancelled, all the stakeholders must be informed well in advance instead of at the last minute—a personal call with apology is preferable to an SMS, which is preferable to an email that may not be read in time leading to misunderstandings all around.

(f) All sessions should preferably be performed only during office hours and that too on workdays; outside of these timings, these should be conducted only for emergencies.

2. At the start of the session, the patient should be warmly greeted, and then ask him to verify his identity to ensure that the correct patient is receiving the consultation.

3. Take his consent next to receive care from a distance after informing him about the details and allaying any fears or concerns that he might have about the teleconsultation—it is preferable to record the entire encounter for medico-legal purposes—the patient should be made aware of this fact with sufficient clarity or else the act of recording itself may constitute a breach of the prevailing laws of the land.

4. Appropriate entries should be made into the EMR throughout the encounter to ensure that as much of necessary information as possible is captured.

5. Patient's EHR must be reviewed and his general progress noted—"how are you doing?" with a smile goes a long way in gaining an instant interpersonal connection and building trust.

6. Interact as necessary; many patients are tech-savvy enough to be able to use their home-based/remote-based devices, while others will benefit from having a carer or a care provider in the form of another clinician or a nurse or a paramedic or even a health worker beside him to help out.

7. The patient should be encouraged to speak and eager relatives or carers gently discouraged from pre-empting them, even when the patient is a young person.

8. The patient's condition should be discussed, informing him about how he is doing clinically and explaining the advice being provided and the why and how of the treatment plan.

(a) If the primary clinician is present, the case should be discussed with him and guidance provided exactly like one would do in all cases of referral.

(b) If any physical examination is required, it must be ensured that this is performed by an appropriately qualified person—the alternative is to ask the patient to come in for an encounter in person as soon as possible.

9. The session should be signed off with a "thank you and have a nice day" message—people appreciate this very much and go a long way in having a positive impact upon patient satisfaction.

10. The records entered in the EMR should be reviewed and digitally signed as necessary.

11. One must only now move on to the next appointment on schedule, repeating the steps from # 2 as above onwards—clinicians will do well to remember to take a 5 min break after every hour of telemedicine consultation; this must be built in to the appointment schedule to help minimise fatigue, both physical and mental.

Setting It Up

It is best to treat the entire teleconsultation venture as a business project. This will ensure that it is handled in a professional manner where mistakes get minimised, if not entirely eliminated, and success rates and long-term viability are maximised.

It is assumed that the telemedicine room has been set up and fully equipped with connectivity between the various locations established, and everything functioning optimally. Setting up a teleconsultation room with all the necessary equipment and connectivity is not a job for amateurs or the "naturally gifted" and must be done by sufficiently experienced professionals. The extra expense incurred on this account is money well spent as it ensures the hassle-free operation of the entire project for which optimally running equipments with robust connectivity are crucial and make the difference between roaring success and utter failure.

Some very successful commercial videoconferencing (including telepresence content collaboration and communication) companies are doing brisk business and have proven ability to provide comprehensive solutions to facilitate the smooth functioning of teleconsultation sessions. Although somewhat expensive, the benefit is that they provide the equipment, set it up, do test runs, perform periodic maintenance and have great after-sales services. All this makes it well worth considering, provided that the price is right.

Since it is expected that most patients will either be in their home or visiting some local facility, ADSL or mobile connectivity is perhaps the best option for the former and MLLN for the latter. This of course means that the clinician's end will have to have provisions for both and this will increase the incurred costs. Telepresence is best delivered through dedicated leased line network as it provides a certain degree of comfort of shielding from snooping, albeit at a price. ADSL-based Internet connections can be used by laptops, tablets and smartphones that have built-in audio-video equipment to facilitate low-cost teleconsultations quite well. Using these for such interactions is quite acceptable and is well worth trying. *In fact, a large part of the cost of goods sold in the* pro forma *I & E for teleconsultation (provided in a later chapter) can be eliminated, thereby significantly bringing down most of capex as well as opex* (Fig. 7.1).

The figure above depicts the teleconsultation ecosystem. The care provider's end (clinician) and the care receiver's end (patient) are interconnected directly (using any suitable telecommunications link like high-speed dedicated leased line, ADSL, 3G/4G/5G, etc.) and indirectly via an EHR system that is preferably Cloud-based. It is worth noting that while there is only one-way connection between the patient and the EHR, there is a two-way connection with the clinician. This is since all the information gathered from the patient get sent to the system while the clinician not only interacts (reviews and queries) with it but also enters his observations into it. The various scanners, monitors and wearables collect clinical data from the patient and send them across both to the EHR system and directly to the clinician, which are then displayed using a variety of display monitors, tablets, computers and printers. The readers should note that the audio-visual equipments have not been displayed at either end to reduce clutter and increase clarity. Nevertheless, they are deemed present.

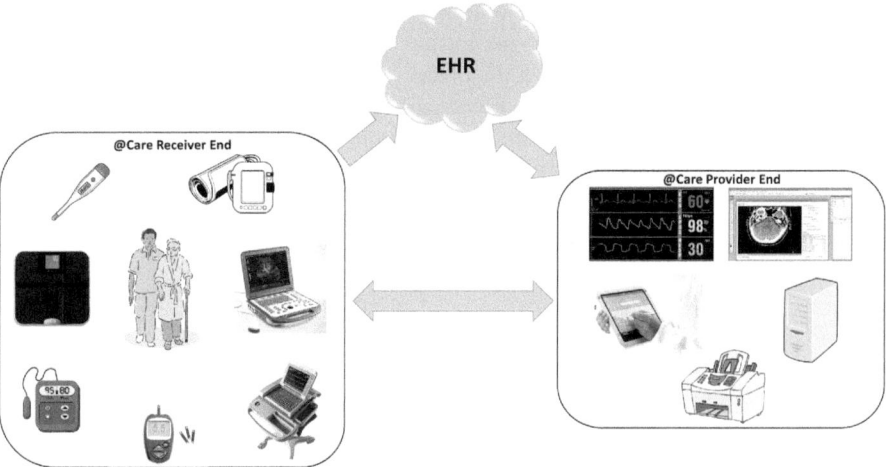

Fig. 7.1 Teleconsultation ecosystem

Running

Most equipment will work as soon as they are powered on. That does not guarantee that they will work fine too. A test run of sorts is always a good idea to ensure that no one is unnecessarily frustrated. If something is not working, it needs to be fixed right away.

Maintenance

Every equipment will require periodic maintenance. An annual maintenance contract is worth it provided it is comprehensive, ideally does not cost more than 10% of the total cost of equipment and has provision for regular check-up as well as attends calls for onsite repairs on demand.

A good process would be to replace old equipment at regular intervals even if they are working alright. Most of the modern equipment tends to become obsolete within 3 years. This factor must always be kept in mind.

Concluding Remarks

Teleconsultation remains and is expected to remain the *de facto* telemedicine service offering. This must be accepted. However, with progressive advancement in technology and consequent availability of better tools, this type of service can be expected to be quite commonplace that is hopefully inexpensive in the near future, almost like the by-now-ubiquitous cellphone.

Many of the currently available and widely used chat messaging applications offer both telephony and video-phony using Internet connection via mobile or broadband—the higher the speed, the better. The only downside to them is the large data bandwidths required by any teleconsultation, and so opting for a higher data plan with high enough speeds remains a wise choice. This makes the possibility of providing no-frills teleconsultations a relatively easy thing to conduct without much fuss.

Telemonitoring

8

Abstract

This chapter provides the details as to how telemonitoring services may be offered to patients. The methodology required and steps for setting the services up, running it and performing maintenance of the various equipments and instruments involved are all discussed.

Overview

As previously explained, telemonitoring is where the care providers, mostly attending consultants and doctors (e.g. all registrars, residents, etc.) who are primarily responsible for treating a patient, are interconnected so that they may attend to the patient 24 × 7, even if "virtually", no matter where they are physically located.

Irrespective of where the patient is physically located in a facility—in critical care, single room or ward—and whether he is ambulatory or on a wheelchair or confined to bed, through this service all of his attending care providers are able to get up-to-date information about the patient's latest health status, no matter what that information might be. They would be able to access the patient's charts (EMRs, EHR) and readouts from monitors and using telepresence interact with the nursing and paramedical staff and the patient irrespective of where they physically are—in their clinics and chambers, on the road, at home, attending a conference in a different city, etc.

Telemedicine technology enables the required information to be available on a variety of platforms like home computers, tablets, smartphones, PDA or other mobility devices. It will be preferable if a single portal or application (including mobility app) is able to provide the entire range of information that can be telemonitored. The ability to interact with the patient and the nursing/paramedical staff accompanying them requires that telepresence facility be also available. Happily,

© Springer Nature Singapore Pte Ltd. 2017   69
S.B. Bhattacharyya, *A DIY Guide to Telemedicine for Clinicians*,
DOI 10.1007/978-981-10-5305-4_8

this is possible by using any of the audio-video chatting and messaging apps that are both readily available and quite popular.

It is expected that once the value of telemonitoring is recognised, sufficient market traction will get generated for the solution vendors to begin offering comprehensive "telemonitoring solutions". (It would not be out of place here to point out that such solutions are already available commercially for the critical care space and those covering other specialities in the pipeline). The only current downside to this are the costs involved, making it a "nice-to-have" feature instead of a "need-to-have" one.

The pro forma I & E calculations for telemonitoring provided in a later chapter demonstrates how telemonitoring can be offered to all admitted patients at zero or near-zero costs. This should be a good reason for all clinicians to seriously think about offering this type of telemedicine service to their patients.

Methodology

The following are the essential steps. Since this is mostly for the clinician's comfort, the patient needs to be accommodated only so far as to ensure they are not inconvenienced in any way.

1. Identifying the patients who need telemonitoring—although only those requiring constant monitoring would be the ideal candidates, the comfort that telemonitoring provides to the involved care providers, especially the busy constantly-on-the-move visiting consultants who may have several of their patients simultaneously admitted in different facilities physically located at a distance from each other, and the relatively easy availability of the necessary telemonitoring equipment makes the possibility of offering telemonitoring services to all admitted patients no challenge worthy of mention.
2. Ensuring that only the essential information is sent through—not every data under the sun being necessary—the physically attending staff can inform everything that is important enough to report (the importance of having properly trained and experienced personnel can neither be overstated nor overemphasised for telemonitoring).
3. Ensuring that continuous access to all medical charts in electronic format including EHR and EMR is available, along with the ability to instantaneously discuss with and issue treatment orders to the attending care providers who are physically present with the patients and receive feedback regarding the various interventions made along with their outcomes is both vital and necessary.
4. Making it a point to "virtually" visit the patient at least once per day even just to say "hello, how are you doing?" with a smile.
5. If the clinician is going to be physically away for more than 24 hours, it is better that the patients are informed about this in person so that they do not get unduly worried; in fact, all attending clinicians should try and visit as often as required, but not too many times within a 24 hours period lest the patients start becoming anxious as to why their doctor is checking up ever so often and begin to wonder whether or not something is seriously wrong with them that necessitates such attention.

6. Interacting with the patients, taking time to inform them about their overall progress and discussing the future course of treatment to give them the feeling that the "virtual" visit is in no way any different from a physical one; informing them "you are doing great" if they are does wonders for patient morale and leads to high levels of patient satisfaction.
7. An attending care provider can perform the required physical examinations and bedside evaluations using various health monitors and biosensors and report back the findings—this person must be trustworthy enough to perform the necessary tasks, and from a legal standpoint, it is preferable for this person to be a qualified and experienced healthcare professional.
8. The general dictum to follow would be to treat the encounter as a "clinical round".
9. Signing off with a "goodbye and see you soon" and a smile.

Setting It Up

Normally the equipments are in continuously running mode as they can be detached from one patient and attached to another without much delay, taking all necessary precautions related to sterilisation and infection control. Patient identification is most crucial—the fact that wrong identities can result in fatalities needs to be borne in mind at all times.

The clinical monitors and biosensors in most instances will need to be connected to their respective aggregating devices that act as base units, which will then need to be connected to the remote units or solutions or apps as required so that the data generated by them get telemetered through seamlessly. When the readouts are recorded in an EMR or verbally informed by the care provider physically attending the patient or the patient himself, using any suitable telecommunications medium like phone, video chat, voice chat, messaging apps, telepresence, etc., that information is available to the clinician in a pretty seamless manner right away in real time.

The clinician should check that everything is in order before leaving the premises. This may involve carrying out a test run, preferably in the presence of the patient, so that both the patient and the clinician are certain that everything is in proper working order. Even if they do not say so, patients (and their relations/carers) are bound to be concerned about the efficacy of the entire telemonitoring process. *This however should decrease over time as the service becomes more commonplace.*

The telemonitoring process must have adequate provisions for carrying out on-demand teleconsultations with or without telepresence. Both the clinician and the patient will derive great satisfaction from being able to see, hear and speak to each other. Since most of the interactions in telemonitoring scenarios are likely to tend to be more "informal" than "formal", high-end equipment is not usually required (although no harm comes from using them), and a chat messaging application running on a PC or a tablet or even a smartphone should prove to be quite acceptable in most situations. The fact that the clinician may be on the move and the connectivity will mostly be through mobile connections must be borne in mind when considering the level of sophistication of the teleconsultation equipment used where the less sophisticated ones are better (Fig. 8.1).

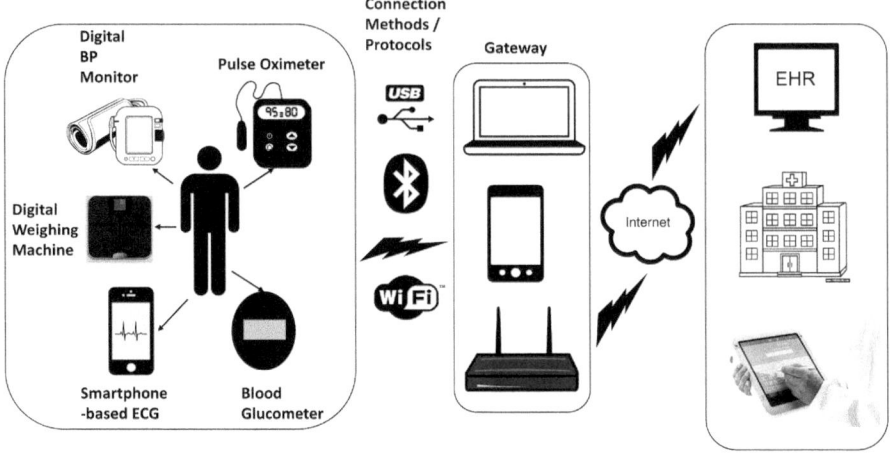

Fig. 8.1   Schematic ecosystem for telemonitoring

The figure above depicts the ecosystem for telemonitoring. Biosensors and monitors at the patient's end collect data both synchronously and asynchronously and use a variety of connection methods and protocols like Bluetooth®, Wi-Fi and even USB memory sticks to telemeter/upload the data to an EHR system or an application in the hand of the clinician using a laptop or smartphone and a suitable router as the gateway to the Internet. Some of the data may be informed over the phone or video chat or messaging app by someone at the patient's end to the clinician—*this has not been depicted to simplify the figure.*

Running It

This is somewhat tricky as one has to decide what all to include and what all to exclude from regular monitoring. A test run for each equipment is required to ensure that everything is working like clockwork.

When the clinician is away and something does not work, it is bound to cause a good deal of frustration, annoyance and even consternation amongst all stakeholders and must therefore be fixed right away. If a critical data item is not being telemetered through, it must be taken care of forthwith for no delay can be brooked at any time—they add to the risk of morbidity and mortality.

Concluding Remarks

Tragically still a much underutilised telemedicine service type, telemonitoring can provide very tangible benefits to both the clinician and the patients under his care. Too frequently a busy clinician is unable to visit all patients under his care due to a variety of reasons. This unfortunately leads to the must-avoid situation where the patient naturally feels abandoned and uncared for even though his bills keep running up. No one can ever be happy with this state of affairs, especially one who is ill and anxious.

A common complaint of many patients is that their doctors do not take good care of them, generally leaving it to be provided by their relatively inexperienced juniors who, in their opinion, are unable to manage their cases optimally. Telemonitoring will go a long way in help addressing this situation.

It will also do everyone a world of good to recognise that poor communication is the cause of most angst amongst the stakeholders and telemonitoring is a great tool to "remain in touch".

Since the clinician remains in charge and is actually merely "checking up" and providing advice regarding the future course of treatment, he is "deemed" to have continued legal responsibility without any further ramifications in this regard, legal or otherwise. Hence, he must exercise due caution as deemed necessary at all times.

Remote Care

9

Abstract

This chapter provides the details as to how remote care services may be offered to patients. The methodology required and steps for setting the services up, running it and performing maintenance of the various equipments and instruments involved are all discussed.

Overview

Rather than continuing to remain largely esoteric, telemedicine services in its newest avatar as remote care, comprising of telehomecare and remote patient monitoring for wellness and preventive care, are quickly transforming the way individuals are being provided care. Instead of patients having to make that extra effort at additional costs to visit their care providers in person just for a review, they can now be informed whether everything is hunky-dory or whether they need to get in touch with their doctor right away, from within the comforts of their homes.

This change is truly transformational and definitely holds the promise of better and affordable care in terms of better outcomes and increased efficiency at reduced costs overall. Without a doubt, remote care holds the promise of being the most exciting innovation in the field of healthcare delivery in general and telemedicine services in particular.

These programmes help the elderly and individuals with health issues to continue living at home instead of being forced to move into facilities where skilled nursing is available. Additionally, they also aid in reducing hospital admissions, readmissions, and stay—all of which help in improving the quality of life overall in a cost-effective manner. By leveraging high-performance computing to provide feedback in real time and using evidence-based medicine, better clinical outcomes can be ensured.

Using healthcare big data analytics and appropriate monitoring systems, clinicians can significantly augment their ability to supervise the health and wellness of the individual and intervene on demand through appropriate alerts/warnings or by asking them to visit a clinician on a priority basis or even making emergency visits for care delivery in a home setting. Measureable benefits of such connected healthcare devices include reduction in mortality rates, clinic visits, emergency admissions and length of inpatient stay. Regulations, use of appropriate healthcare expertise and machine learning are all key success factors for this ecosystem.

Remote Care

As mentioned above, remote care comes in two distinct flavours—telehomecare and remote monitoring. While the former is for people with known illnesses that are mostly chronic in nature requiring close monitoring preferably round the clock, the latter is for health-conscious people who are not otherwise suffering from any illnesses.

It is expected that this particular type of care delivery system would be predominant in the future with the care providers proactively getting in touch with people being monitored just in time when a problem is noted or when a potential for one is discovered so that immediate measures may be initiated before any real problem or a crisis occurs.

Telehomecare

In this telemedicine-enabled homecare setting, digital technologies are used for health data collection from individuals in one location and securely transmitting them to their care providers present in a different location for assessment and making treatment recommendations, *all from within a single digitalised ecosystem.* Such monitoring programmes will collect a wide range of health-related data, such as vital signs, weight, blood sugar, blood oxygen levels, electrocardiograms and even ultrasound scans from the patient, and have these sent across using the Internet, preferably using a VPN to ensure patient-related privacy and confidentiality issues are sufficiently addressed (Fig. 9.1).

The figure above depicts the ecosystem for telehomecare that is aimed towards providing continuous care monitoring services for patients with chronic illnesses. The typical patient who would be the candidates to receive such care services would ideally be a senior citizen living alone or at least who is alone for the greater part of a day, has restricted mobility to varying degrees, is largely housebound and suffers from at least one or more chronic diseases (like diabetes mellitus, hypertension, hypercholesterolaemia, asthma, cardiac arrhythmia with or without intra-cardiac devices like a pacemaker or defibrillator, cancer, etc.) that require evaluation and attention on a continuous basis.

Similar to telemonitoring, the biggest difference here is that all clinical data are collected from a wide variety of monitors and sensors that are either automatically

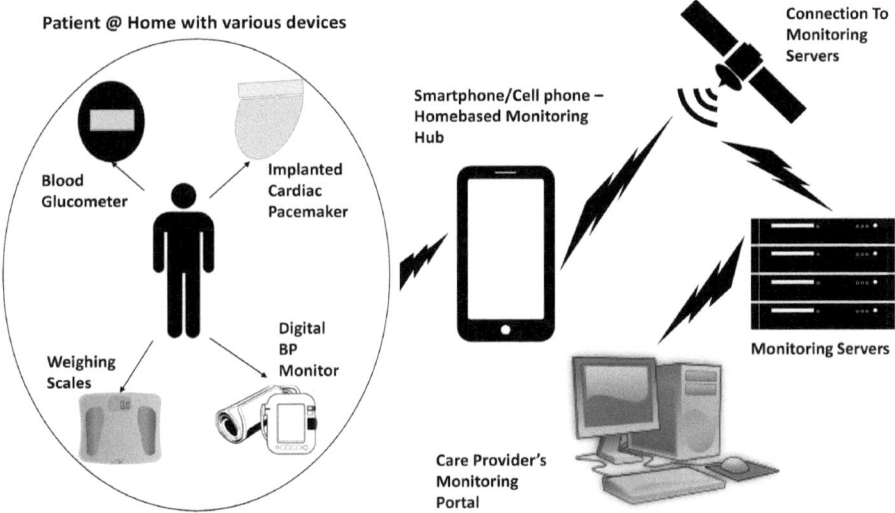

Fig. 9.1 Schematic ecosystem for telehomecare (those with chronic illnesses incl. senior citizens)

telemetered through to or are manually entered into Cloud-based health monitoring servers using a home-based aggregating device that might be a smartphone or a tablet or a dedicated monitoring hub. The remotely located monitoring servers generate reports, alerts and warnings and even initiate automated next steps. Those that would be of interest to the care providers are sent across to the monitoring portals located at their end, while those that require some action to be taken by the patient/ person being monitored are sent to them using their smartphones or similar device including computers. Should the care provider need to call or get in touch with the patient in person, the phone or functionalities like video chat or messaging apps or even telepresence can be used for that purpose.

An imaginary scenario is provided below to help illustrate how exactly *telehomecare* might play out[1].

Diabetes-Hypertension-Hypercholesterolaemia (DHH) Monitoring
Dramatis Personae

1. Cedric—diabetes mellitus type II with hypertension and hypercholesterolaemia sufferer
2. Rebecca—community nurse
3. Rowena—dietician
4. Brian—diabetologist
5. Robin—cardiologist
6. Wilfred—TCIMonitors IT head

---

[1] This is completely imaginary and a work of pure fiction written in the style of use case scenario. Any similarities with an actual case are purely coincidental and totally unintentional.

Scenario

Cedric is a 75-year-old type II diabetic with hypertension and hypercholesterolae-mia. He was diagnosed around 10 years ago and has signed up for continuous moni-toring of his condition by an organisation called The Chronically Ill Monitors, TCIMonitors for short.

He registered at TCIMonitors website on the recommendation of his diabetolo-gist Dr Brian and is attended at his residence by Rebecca, a community nurse. Upon registration, he has downloaded the TCIMA (The Chronically Ill Monitor & Alert) app on to his smartphone. He has also procured an electronic blood glucometer and an electronic blood pressure and pulse oximeter, both of which are capable of trans-mitting readings over wireless using Bluetooth® technology. Wilfred is very helpful in addressing any concerns or queries he has when using the app.

The TCIMA app is capable of the following:

1. Monitoring (through Wi-Fi/Bluetooth®)
   (a) Electronic blood glucose monitors
   (b) Electronic BP and pulse oximeters
   (c) Electronic weighing machines
2. Using the mobile device's capabilities to
   (a) Monitor distance walked per day using GPS and accelerometer
   (b) Monitor spatial location using gyroscope
3. Interacting with individuals to
   (a) Ask diet-related, physical activity-related and general condition-related questions and receive responses
   (b) Inform about diet, drug and physical activity compliance status
   (c) Inform about general physical condition status
   (d) Inform about healthy living/lifestyle status
   (e) Reminders regarding medications related to its name, quantity and the time to take it
   (f) Reminders regarding scheduled home-based and lab testing and appointments
4. Ability to get in touch with a designated community nurse or primary care physi-cian on demand

Every morning Cedric wakes up to find a message reminding him to have his fasting blood glucose level checked. Once he successfully performs the task, the monitor automatically transmits the reading to his TCIMA maintained Cloud-based EHR. The system informs him through a message the interpretation of the result like "Your sugar levels are acceptable this morning" or "Your sugar levels are high this morning. Take two tablets of Drug A with your breakfast. Re-check after 2 hours", etc. He keeps his smartphone on his person as he has his breakfast and takes his other medications. He uses the rear-end camera of his smartphone to take pictures of the various items he has for breakfast. The TCIMA app informs him about the number of calories he has ingested and the balanced number of calo-ries he can take for the rest of the day. He is reminded about the various medica-tions that he needs to take at breakfast, and once he takes them, he clicks a button to indicate that he has indeed complied. If he forgets or misses taking his required medications, he is repeatedly reminded about this. Should he fail to respond, the app uses the central monitoring server to raise appropriate alert to his diabetologist Dr Brian for follow-up action as deemed fit by him.

The app also reminds him about his physical exercise and dietary needs and home/facility/physician chamber-based investigations and appointments by the date and time of day. He is guided to have his blood pressure, pulse rate and partial pressure of oxygen (SpO_2) monitored several times per day in light of the fact that he had a hitherto unexplained fall in his bathroom about a week back. Although the considered opinion was that this was more of an accident due to slippery floors in the bathroom, it was noted then that he was hypotensive as well as hypoglycaemic all through that fateful day.

He is able to interact online with Rebecca, his community nurse, and Rowena, his dietician. Drs Brian and Robin are able to review his clinical parameters and interact with him and even call him in for an in-person consultation in their clinics. The care providers are also able to track his blood pressure, pulse, blood glucose, periodic HbA_{1c} and blood lipid findings over time. They are also able to monitor his medication and lifestyle compliance and suggest course corrections as necessary. Some of these course-corrective measures are automated using a rules engine within the disease management system that automatically guides Cedric to take corrective measures like repeat tests, less medication intake and increased physical activity or to visit the diabetologist on a priority basis. They are able to get in touch with Wilfred for any specialised reports that they might need to provide better care to Cedric.

Remote Monitoring System

Remote monitoring is a technology that enables monitoring of individuals outside of conventional clinical care settings (healthcare facilities and inpatients) and has the potential of increasing access to care and delivery efficiency while decreasing delivery costs. As a type of non-inpatient healthcare services offering that allows a patient to use handheld (mobile) medical devices to perform routine tests and then have the test results electronically sent to a healthcare professional in real time, remote monitoring helps bring care to the receiver instead of the traditional method of having the receiver visit a healthcare facility to receive it. The schematic representation of the ecosystem is provided below (Fig. 9.2).

The figure above depicts the remote monitoring system aimed towards providing wellness and preventive care services. The major difference between this ecosystem and telehomecare discussed in the previous section is that most of the health monitors and sensors utilised here are wearables that the person being monitored needs to wear. This he does because he is a health-conscious individual who believes in wellness and voluntarily opts for preventive care. Since the person is expected to continue to live a normal life and participate in all his usual activities on a daily basis, both his smartphones/handheld devices and wireless routers used to access the Cloud where the remote care monitor servers are located

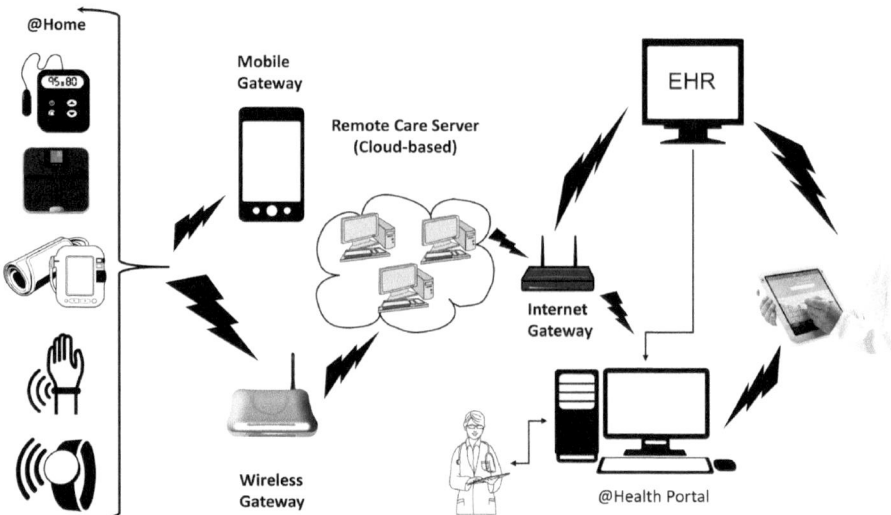

Fig. 9.2 Schematic ecosystem for remote monitoring system (for monitoring health-conscious individuals)

need to be available to him 24×7. The data gets added to the person's EHR so that any care provider would be able to review them on demand using a health portal for that purpose. In case it is necessary to get in touch with the person, the care providers or the monitoring system may do so by using a process that is principally similar to telehomecare.

It is interesting to note that health insurers are already providing incentives in terms of reduced premium rates or higher coverage to those individuals who opt for this type of services. This they are able to do since they can gain confidence in the lifestyle the covered persons lead and predict the most likely health-related issues that might crop up to a very high degree of accuracy—a sort of reward for being a "responsible individual".

It should also be noted here that the remote monitoring system would be the most expensive part of the ecosystem since it needs to not only process all data made available to it but additionally be capable of running big data analytics (since the data will be coming from many individuals who opt to avail such care services, it will almost exclusively be in the form of big data) and raising appropriate messages in the form of alerts and warnings (just as in telehomecare) and passing these on to the person and/or the care provider at the monitoring end.

Such alerts and warnings may be as trivial as "hi, it's time to wake up and go for your morning jog" or "your total calorie intake for the day has exceeded your preset target" to the quite serious "it is well past your usual lunchtime, and you are in danger of missing your midday meal today" or "your heart rate exceeds your limit; please go and lie down immediately" for the person. For the care provider, a different set of alerts and warnings is warranted.

An imaginary scenario is provided below to help illustrate how exactly *remote monitoring for preventive care* might play out[2].

Medication Alerts and Feedback Monitoring
Dramatis Personae

1. Isabelle—patient on regular medication
2. Oliver—community nurse
3. Philip—primary care physician
4. William—regulatory official
5. Shivaram—Good Meds IT head

Jane is a patient on regular medication. She has signed up for medication alerts and feedback by an organisation called Good Meds. She has also procured an electronic BP and pulse monitor that is capable of transmitting readings using wireless communication link.

She registered at Good Meds website on the recommendation of her primary care physician Dr Timothy, and she is attended at her residence by Oliver, a community nurse. Upon registration, she has downloaded the MAF (Medication Alerts and Feedback) app onto her mobile phone. Shivaram is very helpful in addressing any concerns or queries he has when using the app.

Dr Philip has filled in Isabelle's prescription using a CPOE (computerised physician order entry) system along with the various rules, guidelines and possible side effects that Isabelle needs to respectively overlook, be careful about and report if they occur. Oliver, on reviewing it along with Isabelle, has set up the date and times at which Isabelle will take those medications.

Every day the app alerts Isabelle about the medication name, quantity (one tablet, two teaspoonfuls, etc.), the way to take it (swallow, apply, etc.) and the time at which to take. Jane is able to even see what the medication looks like (tablet colour, size, etc.) if she so wishes. After she takes the medication, she clicks a button on the app to indicate she has taken it. If she forgets to take the medication or provide feedback, she is reminded with various modes of alerts—first only onscreen, second with onscreen alert and a beep, third with onscreen alert and several beeps, fourth with automated callback and fifth with alert to Jill and Dr Philip so that Oliver can visit Jane and check on her physically. The time of response or lack thereof is noted for further analysis and recommendations for Dr Philip and Oliver related to patient compliance.

At various times throughout the day, Isabelle is asked to respond through the app by making a choice and clicking a button regarding any ill effects she might be feeling after taking the medication. All information is carefully logged and analysed further by way of signal processing. All reportable adverse events—significant,

---

[2] This is completely imaginary and a work of pure fiction written in the style of use case scenario. Any similarities with an actual case are purely coincidental and totally unintentional.

severe, etc.—are tagged and further analysed and the reports prepared and submitted for further action by the appropriate authorities including Oliver, Dr Philip and William who can get back to Shivaram to seek more detailed analysis and reports about these events.

Hardware Requirements

To provide remote care, the following hardware equipment represents the minimum configuration requirement:

1. Health monitors and biosensors—can be several; term includes all wearables, handheld analysers (like glucometer), mobile monitors, etc.
2. Aggregating home-based hub that can be a smartphone or some dedicated device—for receiving and routing data from monitors and sensors to a remote monitoring server, usually located in the Cloud using VPN or not.
3. Connection to the Cloud—existing high-speed Internet connections can be used via both smartphones and home-based routers.
4. Remote patient monitoring server—this is located at the remote end with a provider keeping a continuous vigil for readouts, alerts and warnings raised from the data received from the biosensors and initiating the necessary interventions on their part; usually located in the Cloud.

Software Requirements

The health monitors, biosensors and central home-based data aggregation devices usually have the necessary software embedded within them. It is the monitoring server that requires specially designed software to be made available. The requirements for these generally would be as follows.

Monitoring Server
The actual networking architecture (central or federated) will depend on the monitoring requirements provided by the facility (more commonly) or individual (rarely)—safer to assume it will be central, i.e. one server connecting to a number of biosensors monitoring patients/person that are either attached to patients or bedside; in most of the cases, the data will qualify as "big data" and will need to cater to the following.

The monitoring server will most likely use the Cloud-based "infrastructure as a service" functionality (discussed in a previous chapter) to perform its various tasks.

1. Gather data from all the connected remote sources continuously on a 24 × 7 (round the clock, every day of the year) basis that will arrive continuously and usually in large amounts.
2. The data will need to be identifiable with the patient as the source of the data, thereby ensuring the accuracy of the data as well as the trustworthiness or reliability of the data source.

3. The data will be of varied types—alphanumeric (text), numerical (floating with decimal places) and binary; image, video and audio types will usually be present in only few instances.
4. Real-time big data analysis.
   (a) Rules for alerts and warnings will be preset for each data item specific to a patient along with the required follow-up action—e.g. if the systolic BP of the patient with unique identification number *1234567890* is more than 140 mmHg, inform the patient through SMS or a chat message sent to the number *XXXXXXXXXX* and/or an email sent to the email address *someone@ somewhere.nnn* with the message "Your blood pressure is high. You are advised to immediately go lie down".
   (b) For each of rules preset above, the server will execute the designated tasks as per the rules.

Methodology

The following are the essential steps:

1. There must be a remote care programme existing and running.
2. Patients (or persons) will need to be enrolled with registration beforehand—they will usually be asked to pay a fee that may be a periodic plan or lump sum as part of a package deal.
3. Consent must compulsorily be taken on enrolment—this is not only a legal requirement but also an ethical necessity. If the patient is unable to provide consent, then his legal representative will need to provide it (this will be more often the case than not as those requiring such continuous monitoring will mostly be senior citizens with chronic conditions who are likely to be living alone or in an active assisted living scenario).
4. The rules for alerts and warnings must be set and subsequently adjusted, preferably in consultation with the attending/primary care physician, the patient and their care providers as well as those who may be attending on them, as and when required.
5. A test run must be carried out to ensure that everything is in working order.
   (a) This should be done after the devices have been set up and connected through to the monitoring server.
   (b) Training sessions for the patient, their carers and anyone else involved should be carried out at this stage so that each stakeholder is fully aware of when to do what to ensure everything runs like clockwork.
   (c) Periodic test runs and retraining sessions must be planned and carried out to ensure that things are proceeding according to plan, and in case any shortcomings are noted, these should be immediately addressed and necessary tweaking of the rules and responses undertaken without delay.
6. The remote monitoring should be initiated—a contact number, preferably toll free, should be provided to the patient and their carers to get in touch 24 × 7 should the need arise, health related or otherwise.

Setting It Up

The health monitors and biosensors, most of which will be in the form of wearables, should be attached and used as required. Patients and their carers may need training to put them on and off, change power supply/batteries and connect through to the monitoring servers using the required aggregation devices and routers. The monitoring servers will also need to be checked to ensure that the data is indeed getting telemetered through (this will be a part of the test run mentioned in the previous section).

Running It

Identifying the "right" candidates to receive such care is required since not every patient needs such close attention even though they may want it. This choice must however be need based and not based on their ability to pay for the service. Manipulating or forcing someone to opt for such services would be blatantly unfair and should be construed as an instance of unethical practice.

Periodic teleconsultations and actual physical visits made to the patient's premises occasionally must be carried out to provide the necessary assurances to all the concerned stakeholders that things are indeed going according to plan.

Concluding Remarks

Remote care is still somewhat futuristic and is expected to remain so for a few more years at least. However, some basic form of remote monitoring where a patient, attached to only a single device, is continuously monitored remotely may not be that esoteric in the very near future.

Needless to say, with the increasing number of seniors living longer—the silver tsunami—many with chronic conditions, and alone, this mode of monitoring can be expected to become increasingly the norm rather than the exception.

When the need for addressing wellness and preventive care issues is concerned, particularly in context of increased health consciousness and raised awareness about benefits of adhering to a healthy lifestyle backed up with careful monitoring, this mode of monitoring can be expected to be increasingly sought after.

To be prepared for such eventualities will definitely be wise and make perfect business sense for all the concerned stakeholders.

Abstract

This chapter discusses the management aspects involved in offering telemedicine sessions. Examples of income and expenditure calculations have been provided with brief financial analysis for the three types of telemedicine services that this DIY guide deals with, namely, teleconsultations, telemonitoring and remote care.

Overview

Although taking a professional approach when considering whether to offer any of the telemedicine services by individual clinicians may feel like to be bit of an overkill, it proves to be wiser in the long run. Nothing can be easier to use a feature or an app already available in one's smart device for telemedicine without much of a forethought. Should one wish to just "remain in touch" using the technology, then this should be sufficient in most cases. However, if one wishes to use it for anything more than just being "with the times", adoption of sound management techniques early on provides more positives than not.

A few management home truths *(the following have been provided without prejudice)*:

- All business are run to create wealth, i.e. to be profitable, where income exceeds expenditure. If charitable, all monies lent do not usually have to be repaid, taxes are usually exempted and all profits are ploughed back into the business. If not-for-profit, only the profits are ploughed back into the business, but all interests and taxes have to be paid. If for-profit, the business must make a profit as the shareholders or owners expect to earn from it. So, if the pro forma I & E does not reveal profits, one must not even think about running that line of business.
- Finance ensures one survives till tomorrow. Strategy ensures one survives till next year. Strategic vision is more important than financial gain.

- Short-term financial compromises are okay if they ensure long-term strategic success.
- Free cash flow is the most important thing. Nothing beats cash in hand.
- Yesterday was a dream. Today is a reality. Tomorrow is a hope.
- Administration is proactive, performed by leaders and concerned more with the overall vision, while management is reactive, performed by followers and concerned more with the implementation aspects.
- Plans need to be practical; it isn't good enough if it remains only on paper.
- When booking profits, one must always be ever vigilant against the very human predilection of giving in to greed. One mustn't kill the golden goose that lays golden eggs; instead, one must carefully nurture it.
- Convert every question mark into a star, every star to a cash cow, and suitably handle your dogs to keep competitors out (*refer to BCG matrix components*).
- Discipline in every aspect is of the essence. Lose it and lose the business.
- Assess risk, then take it or forsake it.
- Analyse impact, then do what is best for one's business.

An Important Note

It is possible to create a business model where services are provided on a "no-cost-to-consumer" basis. Tricky, yes, but very much possible. Taking such a decision represents a long-term vision instead of short-term one.

The revenues in such a scenario need to accrue from indirect sources – the so-called "soft" factors. This could be increased customer satisfaction leading to increased goodwill that in turn leads to increased awareness amongst potential customers that finally leads to increased consumer volumes culminating in increased revenues from other services rendered to them representing a healthy return on investment in the medium to long term.

Due to various reasons related to maintenance and upgrades, the "free" model is often found not to be sustainable in the long run. Hence, anyone planning to offer this, for whatever reason, needs to make careful financial assessments first before even thinking of going ahead.

Alternatively, it could also be made a part of the overall care delivery services where the costs incurred and the additional revenues expected from are factored into the care service offering mix. An example of this would be to offer it to every patient either as part of their consultation or inpatient's stay or at a special rate that may be charged specifically for the extra services rendered.

Done properly, it additionally translates into increased consumer volumes, although the increased volume may not be as high as a "free" service as many consumers may balk at the need to pay extra. Also, creating a mechanism where some consumers use the premium service that aids in the delivery of better care and contribute positively to better outcomes, while the rest who opt not to but suffer as a consequence may lead to avoidable frictions within the system that may be detrimental to the business overall. Droves of aggrieved consumers are worse than a wake of vultures feeding on a not-yet-dead animal, and that scenario can definitely never be good for business.

Business Model

A business model is the way in which a company expects to generate revenue and make profit from company operations. A good business model will ensure that the business is an overall success in terms of revenues, profits, further investments and growth, thereby making it a reasonably acceptable risk to go into – both for the investor and the business sponsor/owner alike.

Business Case

Let us assume that a clinician observes that offering telemedicine services to patients under his care would be useful for his practice. He needs to first decide what services all to offer. This would generally be based on his interactions with his patients and staff. Once he decides to offer either one or several different types of services, he needs to figure out whether he needs to set up a company to do that or extend the service offerings of his existing practice. In case of the former, he would need to have a business plan and in the latter a business case prepared to help convince his investors (usually the dear old and hopefully cooperative bank manager) to cough up the necessary dough required to fund it.

For example, while a hospital would perhaps be interested to provide teleconsultation or telemonitoring and hence will prepare a business case to support it, a clinician will need to prepare a business plan. For remote care, it would more often be the case that a business plan would be required since such specialised services can only best be offered by a new company.

In either case, the output document is principally for the investors or creditors (financers, banks and sundry lenders).

One needs to make a cool and calculated decision that one wants to offer a particular set of telemedicine services. One must then collect sufficient justification for that decision before deciding on the range of services that one plans to offer. Only then should one go ahead and take the plunge. The following questions help in the process.

1. What's in it for me?
2. How will it benefit me and my business?
3. What all tools are required for this?
4. Where can I source them from?
5. How much will it cost to set everything up?
6. Who all can help me?
7. Do I need a place to run it from? If yes, where should I locate it? Why that particular place? How do I acquire, fund and run it?
8. What all changes do I need to make in my current business in terms of
   (a) Infrastructure
   (b) Personnel
   (c) Work processes

The business case/plan document is for the proposer (of the business) repre-senting his strategic vision. Its aim is to provide sufficient guidance to him on his journey towards meeting his business objectives – the reason for him taking the plunge instead of investing in the money market and relax as he watches his money grow.

The target audience for the document however are the investors or creditors (financers, banks and sundry lenders) representing the financial aspects of the busi-ness – how much it will cost, how much profit is expected, etc. – all supported with facts, figures, analysis, reports, charts and graphs. Its aim is to provide sufficient evidence for the lenders to have confidence in the business venture.

Profit and loss is calculating profit or loss that is expected from the business and the projections are usually made for either 3 or 5 years. All are best-guess estimates (aka best guess-estimates) since these are projections. It is wise to have two estimates of both the volumes and the revenues – optimistic (high) and pessimistic (low) – to figure out whether it is wiser to invest in or mark it as a "no go" based on the financial assessments. One must also always be mindful of the value of "goodwill". This intangible item proves to be a key success factor of any business venture quite often.

Usually a business case/plan will generally be expected to have the following sections.[1] Suffice it to say, its preparation is best left to experienced professionals, and the cost incurred thereof is money well spent.

- Executive summary
- Introduction and overview
- Current market analysis (with gaps identified)
- Cost-benefit analysis
- Options evaluation
- Key assumptions and dependencies
- Risk and sensitivity analysis
- Resource requirements and cost
- Pro forma income and expenditure statement (3 or 5 year[2] projection with NPV and IRR calculation – mention the WACC/interest (hurdle) rate considered)
- Project timelines (estimated)
- Conclusions
- Recommendations

---

[1] List inspired by a Business Case Template made available by National Innovation Centre, NHS, UK

[2] Although 5 years is the norm, for all projects that are IT-related or have a heavy IT component, it is wiser to have a 3 year projection to factor in the rapid changes in the underlying technologies that might impact the project by rendering existing systems (both hardware and software) obsolete.

Costing Telemedicine Services

Being a service, the various components need to include the "human" factors like goodwill of the person/persons performing the service, cost of their training (including retraining), salary/consultation fees to be paid, etc. The time taken to provide the service, connection charges, etc. needs to be calculated also. Although paid periodically, they behave as fixed costs for all effective purposes as they generally tend to remain the same. Furthermore, being a service, it has no inventories. This is both a good thing and a bad thing: good, because no inventory carrying costs are incurred; bad, because the services cannot be stored for future use and need to be produced at the time of consumption. When there is no sale, there is no revenue, and periods without sale, which in this case is equivalent to non-utilisation, are lean periods where the fixed costs remain unrecovered.

Analysis

Costing of telemedicine services is, as with most costing exercises, not simple. The various costs of goods sold components of services consist broadly of the equipment used for delivering the services and the human resources utilised to providing them.

Cost Heads

These are the various groupings of cost-incurring items. For telemedicine services, these would be as follows:

1. Fixed
   (a) Equipment
       - Hardware – requires servicing and replacement, but IT-related ones can be depreciated at a faster rate
       - Software – requires periodically recurring licensing fees, upgrading and maintenance
   (b) Salary paid to service providers who are full-time employees (FTE)
   (c) Cost of training and retraining personnel
   (d) Office furniture
2. Variable
   (a) Running costs
       - Electricity consumed
       - Office rental
       - Office supplies
       - Others
   (b) Cost of goods sold (COGS) – *aka cost of services delivered*
       - Telecommunication connectivity costs

- Consultant costs (for teleconsultations only) – paid either on the number of consultations or number of hours or per diem basis
- Salary paid to contractual workers who typically are paid on an hourly basis for the number of hours actually worked

Cost Drivers

These drive the incurred costs.

Since there are no inventories in services, the cost drivers applicable to telemedicine services are as follows:

1. Number of teleconsultations/telemonitoring sessions undertaken or remote care subscribers
2. Amount of time spent in providing the consultations
3. Length of idle time (*period of no activity*)
4. Length of downtime (*due to any factor*)
5. Turnaround time (TAT) between two sessions

Activity-based costing method is the best. When there is no service to be provided, the variable costs are not incurred. The amount of time spent in providing the services and the idle/downtime are the principle cost drivers.

While the number of sessions is also a cost driver, the length of time taken to perform such consultations and TAT can vary. It will also be necessary to ensure zero or near-zero downtime (six sigma approach would be a good practice to follow) and cut down on idle time to ensure optimal performance.

Although when marginal costs match marginal prices, profit maximisation occurs, it must be noted that whenever the load factor for service delivery exceeds 80%, the service quality usually suffers more often than not. This almost invariably leads to negatively impacting the company's top line and loss of that all-important "goodwill".

Pricing Telemedicine Services

Pricing services is a tricky business. Services are quite unique in nature as they are rendered and tend to be much individualised. They have no shelf-life and they cannot be put into any inventory. They are delivered by a person or a group thereof to a person or a group thereof. So, at what price point is it "just about right" and not become too much? What is the threshold for too little? Should one have a fixed price for all or a flexible one where different rates are offered to different customers based on negotiations with them? These are amongst the many imponderables when deciding prices.

Several pricing methods can be used to price products.[3] These are cost oriented like cost plus pricing, markup pricing, break-even pricing, target return pricing and early cash recovery pricing or market oriented like perceived value pricing, going-rate pricing (are of two types, namely, competitor's 'parity' pricing and premium pricing), discount pricing, sealed-bid pricing and differentiated pricing (that are of four distinctive types, namely, customer segment pricing, time pricing, area pricing and product form pricing).

Cost plus markup or break-even pricing method is an easy method to adopt and works decently enough for telemedicine services with the former returning a profit on every session while the latter ensuring that there is no loss (pricing is supposed to guarantee a no-profit-no-loss).

To price telemedicine services, it is necessary to decide first what the aim of providing it in the first place is. Is it to benefit the consumers? Is it to benefit the providers? Is it for a bit of both? Since profit maximisation occurs when marginal income = marginal cost, should one try and aim for that? Is that morally defensible in healthcare that has a very strong social aspect to it?

A wise way to go about this would be to consider how much it costs to render the service in the first place and then add a "reasonable markup" in order to book the desired profits. This "reasonable" markup is the trickiest bit by far. If there are no competitors, it is possible to get away with a huge number, else one may have to opt for a break-even pricing where only the costs are recovered. Goodwill is an important consideration too for any pricing decision.

The price sensitiveness of the customers and their ability to pay is also an important factor that needs careful consideration. If they are unable to pay the charges, they will not opt for the service in the first place, which results in rendering the entire business model unviable from the very beginning. This feature results in customers balking at any charge they consider to be overpriced. Estimating the demand for services is a good measure to figure out which price is right.

Normally, patients would prefer telemedicine to be available as a free service. Thus, including it as part of an overall package may be wiser and accordingly charged or not. For example, there is a charge for every consultation. If that is charged irrespective of whether it was "in person" or "from a distance", then there should not be much of a problem and the patients accepting it with the least amount of fuss.

Do note that most insurance companies will not defray charges for receiving telemedicine services, although this has begun to change of late.

For remote care, it is wiser to bundle all charges together as a package deal since it includes remote monitoring, teleconsultations and attending in person that cannot be properly segregated as these are rendered on a continuous basis as part of the overall service.

---

[3] Methods of Pricing: Cost-Oriented Method and Market-Oriented Method by Smriti Chand (www.yourarticlelibrary.com/marketing/pricing/methods-of-pricing-cost-oriented-method-and-market-oriented-method/32311/)

Pro forma I & E

This is a financial statement that summarises the revenues earned and the different costs and expenses incurred. *Do note that it is a part of financial management and represents a projection,* i.e. *a forecast, and does not reflect actual numbers, which is part of accounting.*
The various account heads for calculating this are typically as follows.

Earnings

Usually, this is

$$\text{unit price} \times \text{sales volume}$$

In a healthcare delivery services setting, it will be

$$\text{price of all services rendered} \times \text{total number of patients served}$$

and

$$\text{price of all products (investigation, medications, etc.)} \times$$
$$\text{total number of items sold (tests performed, medication dispensed, etc.)}$$

COGS

Aka cost of sales (of services)
Cost of goods sold is the set of direct costs that are incurred during the course of producing the goods (or services) that are eventually sold by a company. This amount includes the cost of all the different materials used to create the goods along with the direct labour costs used to produce them.
To calculate the cost of telemedicine services rendered, one must remember to include the various staff salaries, establishment costs in terms of rent, electricity, water and connectivity costs (could be fixed or per use or a mixture of these two).

EBIT

Earnings before interests and taxes represents how much the business has earned before paying whatever that is compulsorily owed in terms of interests and taxes. It is a measure of how good the management is doing from a business perspective and represents the "true" profits and helps answer such questions as follows: Are the sales efforts satisfactory? Are the products (services) priced correctly, i.e. the paying customers neither are being overcharged nor undercharged? Are the costs under control?

EAT

Earnings after taxes, aka NI or net income, are the "true" income of the business. Do note that the more the better is not always a good thing for it could mean that the management is merely being able to exploit favourable conditions that may or may not last for long.

Cash Flow Analysis

This is a little tricky and requires some degree of understanding the various principles involved plus considerable amounts of practise.

A business is considered to be doing great when it is able to make more cash available to itself as reflected in the account books as "cash in hand" (usually in the bank as liquid cash but free from any liabilities and available for immediate withdrawal). It is worth noting here that this includes cash that is owed to others but is lying with the business due to its accounts payable (this should be as high as possible) and also early payment of sums owed to it by others, i.e. its accounts receivable (this should be as low as possible). It is also necessary to add back all depreciation values since they only represent a bookable expenditure permitted under income tax rules and no actual cash outflow takes place (represents "free air").

NPV

Net present value is the value of the total investment (present value of the estimated cash inflows minus the present value of the estimated cash outflows) as on current date calculated at the current rate of inflation (or WACC). This index is helpful to figure out whether it is worthwhile to make the investment, i.e. assess financial risk of a business as on today. By suitably tweaking the various items, like capital and operational expenditures, and rejigging the income, it is possible to figure out at what point the business may be made viable, if not worthwhile. This "tweaking" should however be done with great care since too much of this is a sure recipe for disaster.

Examples

Special Note: the following examples have been provided purely for illustrative purposes and are meant to demonstrate the attractiveness, or not, of a particular offering. These must in no way to be taken as indicative in any manner or form. It must also be noted that the various costs (capex and opex), volumes and levied charges have been calculated using very realistic figures as prevailing in India in April 2017.

Readers will additionally take note that the currency used is Indian Rupees (₹) and are in multiples of thousands (000 s). For reference purposes, in April 2017 the prevailing conversion rate was USD ($) 1.00 = ~INR (₹) 65.00 (i.e. one US dollar was equal to around sixty-five Indian rupees) or in other words, ₹ 1.00 = ~$ 0.015 (one Indian rupee was equivalent to roughly one and a half US cents).

Teleconsultation
It is assumed that the clinician (or hospital) providing the services will maintain both the patient's and clinician's ends as well as any connectivity costs between the two.

High End: Utilises the Best-of-Breed Equipments
Assumptions

1. Establishment costs:
   (a) Room rent
   (b) Power supply
   (c) Network connectivity
   (d) Air-conditioning
   (e) Lighting
2. Equipments required:
   (a) Both clinician's and patient's ends:
      - Video equipment:
        – High-end camera
        – Ultra HD LED TV screen 50″+
      - Audio equipment:
        – Multidirectional wireless microphone
        – Speakers
      - Furniture – chairs
   (b) Clinician's end:
      - Cloud-based EHR system with electronic prescription module or CPOE integrated with the EMR component – the cost related to this item is expected to be charged on a fixed monthly basis and considered along with the room rent, power supply and network connectivity costs
      - Monitors:
        – Video display screen
        – Image display – DICOM viewer
      - Furniture – tables (for equipments)
   (c) Patient's end:
      - Medical devices
      - Medical scanning equipment – to be used by non-clinical staff who are guided by the remotely located consultant
      - Medical monitors
      - Furniture – table (for positioning/examining patients)

3. Resources:
   (a) Video cameraman
   (b) Audio handler
   (c) Consultant (clinician's end)
   (d) Nurse/technician (patient's end)
4. All costs to be incurred by the facility providing telemedicine consultation, roughly comes to:
   (a) Capex = ₹ 3,000,000.00
   (b) Opex = ₹ 1,200,000.00 per annum
   (c) Leased line costs = ₹ 2,000,000.00 per annum
   (d) Consultant fee (payable per encounter) = ₹ 1,000.00
5. Teleconsultation charges = ₹ 3,500.00 per encounter, irrespective of duration, charge rising by 10% yearly from Year 2
6. Expected number of consultations:
   (a) First year = 75 per month (roughly translates to 3 encounters per working day of each week)
   (b) Yearly growth:
      • Second year of operations = 100%
      • Third year of operations = 50%
      • Fourth year of operations = 25%
      • Year-on-year growth from fifth year of operations = 20%
7. Opex costs to rise 10% year on year
8. AMC = 10% of Capex per year
9. Depreciation = 20% per year, no replacements have been considered within the 5 year calculation period
10. Applicable income tax rate (consolidated) = 33%:
    (a) No tax to be paid if losses are booked for the applicable year.
    (b) No losses are carried over to the following year.
11. Applicable WACC (cost of borrowing) = 6.25% (prevailing rate of interest April 2017) (Table 10.1).

Low End
Assumptions

1. Establishment Costs:
   (a) Room rent
   (b) Power supply
   (c) Network connectivity
   (d) Air-conditioning
   (e) Lighting
2. Equipments required:
   (a) Both clinician's and patient's ends:
      • Laptops – high end
      • Video equipment

Table 10.1 Pro forma I & E for teleconsultation (high end)

Teleconsultation						
All figures ₹ 000's	Year 0	Year 1	Year 2	Year 3	Year 4	Year 5
Volume calculations		900	1800	2700	3375	4050
Charges (per teleconsultation session)		3.5	3.85	4.235	4.6585	5.12435
Salary costs		(1200)	(1320)	(1452)	(1597)	(1757)
Consultants fees		(1)	(1)	(1)	(1)	(1)
Total consultants fees		(900)	(1980)	(3267)	(4492)	(5930)
Yearly room rent, power, connectivity, EHR costs		(3200)	(3520)	(3872)	(4259)	(4685)
I & E statement						
Income	0	3150	6930	11,435	15,722	20,754
Loans (for capital expenditures)	(3000)	0	0	0	0	0
COGS	0	(5600)	(7120)	(8891)	(10,649)	(12,672)
Depreciation	0	(600)	(600)	(600)	(600)	(600)
EBIT	0	(3050)	(790)	1944	4474	7482
Interest costs	0	(538)	(633)	(743)	(853)	(979)
Payable IT	0	0	0	(396)	(1195)	(2146)
EAT	0	(3588)	(1423)	804	2426	4357
Free cash flow	(3000)	(2988)	(822)	1404	3026	4957
NPV @ 6.25%	626					
IRR	9%					

- Inbuilt web camera
- Large display screen attached to laptop display
- Furniture – chairs
(b) Clinician's end:
- Audio equipment:
  - Lapel microphone
  - Headphones
- Cloud-based EHR system with electronic prescription module or CPOE integrated with the EMR component – the cost related to this item is expected to be charged on a fixed monthly basis and considered along with the room rent, power supply and network connectivity costs
- Furniture – tables (for equipments)
(c) Patient's end:
- Audio equipment:
  - Multidirectional microphone – attached to laptop
  - Speakers – attached to laptop
- Medical devices, only portable scanning machines used, if at all
- Medical monitors
- Furniture – table (for positioning/examining patients)
3. Resources:
  (a) Consultant (clinician's end)
  (b) Nurse/technician (patient's end)

4. All costs to be incurred by the facility providing telemedicine consultation, roughly comes to:
    (a) Capex = ₹ 2,000,000.00
    (b) Opex = ₹ 600,000.00 per annum (includes connectivity costs)
    (c) Consultant fee (payable per encounter) = ₹ 1,000.00
5. Teleconsultation charges = ₹ 2,500.00 per encounter, irrespective of duration, charge rising by 10% yearly from Year 2.
6. Expected number of consultations:
    (a) First year = 50 per month (roughly translates to two encounters per working day of each week)
    (b) Yearly growth:
        • Second year of operations = 100%
        • Third year of operations = 50%
        • Fourth year of operations = 25%
        • Year-on-year growth from fifth year of operations = 20%
7. Opex costs to rise 10% year on year.
8. AMC = 10% of Capex per year.
9. Depreciation = 20% per year, no replacements have been considered within the 5 year calculation period.
10. Applicable income tax rate (consolidated) = 33%:
    (a) No tax to be paid if losses are booked for the applicable year.
    (b) No losses are carried over to the following year.
11. Applicable WACC (cost of borrowing) = 6.25% (prevailing rate of interest April 2017).
12. EMI costs have not been considered when calculating free cash flows (Table 10.2).

Discussion and Analysis

In case of high-end teleconsultations, although the NPV[4] is acceptable (as is the IRR[5]), the main problems lie in the need to have high number of cases from the very first day of operation, which may be very ambitious in itself, with the requirement for high capital expenditures being an additional cause for concern.

The figures for low-end teleconsultations do not appear to make any exciting news either. The continued need to have a high number of cases from day one and keep on charging them a high fee remains a matter of concern, although the requirements of capital expenditures (capex) are much more manageable.

All in all, teleconsultation faces challenges from high capex and high volume requirements from the very first day of operations. Since not all patients will require teleconsultation and many would be put off by the charges, which may be several times of a physical face-to-face consultation, coupled with the need for patients to still travel, the target volumes will continue to present signification challenges on a continued basis.

---

[4] Net present value

[5] Internal rate of return

Table 10.2 Pro forma I & E example for teleconsultation (low end)

Teleconsultation						
All figures ₹ 000's	Year 0	Year 1	Year 2	Year 3	Year 4	Year 5
Volume calculations		600	1200	1800	2250	2700
Charges (per teleconsultation session)		2.5	2.75	3.025	3.3275	3.66025
Salary costs		(600)	(660)	(726)	(799)	(878)
Consultants fees		(1)	(1)	(1)	(1)	(1)
Total consultants fees		(600)	(1320)	(2178)	(2995)	(3953)
Yearly room rent, power, connectivity, EHR costs		(1200)	(1320)	(1452)	(1597)	(1757)
I & E statement						
Income	0	1500	3300	5445	7487	9883
Loans (for Capital Expenditures)	(1000)	0	0	0	0	0
COGS	0	(2500)	(3400)	(4456)	(5491)	(6688)
Depreciation	0	(200)	(200)	(200)	(200)	(200)
EBIT	0	(1200)	(300)	789	1796	2994
Interest costs	0	(219)	(275)	(341)	(406)	(481)
Payable IT	0	0	0	(148)	(459)	(830)
EAT	0	(1419)	(575)	300	932	1684
Free cash flow	(1000)	(1219)	(375)	500	1132	1884
NPV @ 6.25%	204					
IRR	9%					

Telemonitoring
Assumptions

1. Telemonitoring service is provided to all admitted patients once a day in a 75-bedded facility with around 80% occupancy; this translates into a total of $75 \times 0.8 \times 365 = 21,900$ telemonitoring sessions rendered per year.
2. Telemonitoring is charged @ ₹25.00 per session.
3. All devices, scanners, etc., already are networking ready, which means that they can be connected via a gateway to the Internet; where monitors and other devices cannot telemeter their data (streaming and non-streaming) through to the remotely located clinician, the data will be entered into a Cloud-based EHR; alternatively, the monitors can be viewed directly by appropriately placing the video cameras or using far-end camera control (wherever possible).
4. No extra resources required specific to telemonitoring.
5. Cloud-based EHR system already in use by the institutions will be used for every admitted patient.
6. Telemonitoring-specific equipment required – facility end.

(a) Laptop or tablet or smartphone that has video chatting or telepresence software installed with suitably located inbuilt video camera(s) and microphone with speakers; the laptops can be placed on mobile trolleys (with castors) and turned around to face towards or away from the patient or towards a specific area or monitor or nursing and paramedical staff as necessary; wherever possible far-end camera control can be used as necessary by the clinician.

(b) Furniture to house far-end camera control-enabled audio-visual unit with castors (nursing trolleys are usually sufficient enough) so that they can be moved about to permit the clinician to view the patient from various sides.

7. Telemonitoring-specific equipment required – clinician's end; it is expected that the modern-day clinician will already be having the following equipment and *will not be incurring extra costs specifically due to telemonitoring*:

(a) Display monitors attached to laptops with HD web camera

(b) Lapel microphone – can be used in tablet/smartphone if so required (this can be a microphone and earphone combo)

(c) Stereophonic noise-cancellation headphone or earphone – can be used in tablet/smartphone if so required (this can be a microphone and earphone combo)

(d) Tablet/smartphone with HD camera – both front and rear

(e) Printer – Wi-Fi networked colour inkjet/laser

8. Opex costs to rise 10% year on year.

9. AMC = 10% of Capex per year.

10. Depreciation = 20% per year, no replacements have been considered within the 5 year calculation period.

11. Applicable income tax rate (consolidated) = 33%:

(a) No tax to be paid if losses are booked for the applicable year.

(b) No losses are carried over to the following year.

12. Applicable WACC (cost of borrowing) = 6.25% (prevailing rate of interest April 2017).

13. There are no EMI costs incurred for any item.

14. Telemonitoring fee to be charged on a per-patient basis, rising at 10% yearly from Year 2 onwards (Table 10.3).

Discussion and Analysis

Looking at the figures above, it is pretty mindboggling that no one has yet considered this aspect of telemedicine seriously. Even by charging ₹ 25.00 (Rupees twenty five only!) as one-time fee on admission, telemonitoring can be provided at a profit from the first year of operations itself. This is a story in itself for sure.

Quite frankly, the facility can choose to offer this service at no cost to the patient and consider all costs incurred specifically due to telemonitoring as sunk costs. The goodwill generated will surely be worth more than what money can buy.

Table 10.3 Pro Forma I&E example for telemonitoring

Telemonitoring						
All figures ₹ 000's	Year 0	Year 1	Year 2	Year 3	Year 4	Year 5
Volume calculations		21900	21900	21900	21900	21900
Charges (telemonitoring for entire inpatients stay – admission to discharge)		0.025	0.028	0.030	0.033	0.037
I & E statement						
Income	0	548	602	662	729	802
Loans (for capital expenditures)	(150)	0	0	0	0	0
COGS	0	(65)	(65)	(65)	(65)	(65)
Depreciation	0	(30)	(30)	(30)	(30)	(30)
EBIT	0	453	507	567	634	707
Interest costs	0	(13)	(13)	(13)	(13)	(13)
Payable IT	0	(145)	(163)	(183)	(205)	(229)
EAT	0	294	331	371	416	464
Free cash flow	(150)	324	361	401	446	494
NPV @ 6.25%	1434					
IRR	226%					

Remote Care
Assumptions

1. Subscription-based model – all marketing- and sales-related costs are sunk costs.
2. Starting off with 100 subscribers in the first month of operations, the service provider adds 100 more every month during the entire 5-year period.
3. All costs incurred at the patient's end to be paid for at cost by the patient and hence not considered.
4. Remote clinician establishment costs:
    (a) Room rent
    (b) Power supply
    (c) Network connectivity
    (d) Air-conditioning
    (e) Lighting
5. Equipment required at the clinician's end:
    (a) Furniture
        • Table to house all the equipment
        • Chairs for monitoring personnel
    (b) Monitors – HD computer screens
    (c) Laptop with HD camera, microphone and speakers
    (d) Health portal
    (e) EHR system
6. Remote monitoring system – specially designed and developed for the facility, hosted in the Cloud:

(a) Cloud hosting costs – paid all upfront annually.

(b) Remote monitoring software – this will collect data from remotely located persons and run data analytics on it to raise automated alerts and warnings for providers as well as monitored persons for further actions and interventions to be initiated as necessary. *This is expected to be custom-built for the service provider and will be Cloud hosted. Needless to say, this is expected to be the single-most expensive piece of equipment used to provide remote care service.*

7. Resources:
   (a) Remote care monitoring personnel
   (b) Care provider (nurse, community nurse, paramedics or health worker) for contacting patient including home visits – one care provider for every ten subscribers

8. Opex costs to rise 10% year on year.

9. AMC = 10% of Capex per year.

10. Depreciation = 20% per year (no replacements have been considered within the 5 year calculation period).

11. Applicable income tax rate (consolidated) = 33%:
    (a) No tax to be paid if losses are booked for the applicable year.
    (b) No losses are carried over to the following year.

12. Applicable WACC (cost of borrowing) = 6.25% (prevailing rate of interest April 2017).

13. There are no EMI costs incurred for any item (Table 10.4).

Discussion and Analysis

Nota Bene: *Considering that with estimates of around 47% of 323 million people in India are senior with at least one chronic disease[6], a remote clinician organisation can reasonably expect to generate sufficient sales (both volumes and income-wise). Consequently, the figures mentioned in the calculations above are not all that unrealistic.*

The financial calculations above, although illustrative, do appear to point towards the reasonable viability of a remote care project that is offered at very modest charges (₹ 3,000.00 i.e. Rupees three thousand only per month) and adding only 100 new subscribers to existing ones every month. This latter figure can certainly be made much higher and should be strived for. *Quite honestly, at such ridiculous low charges and for the benefits offered, 24 × 7 tracking, immediate feedback regarding missed medications or need to get an investigation done or go visit a facility, proactive home visit by a qualified clinician (usually a nurse or a paramedic), etc., if the marketing and sales department are unable to add a whole lot more, they should be changed forthwith by a more competent group of people.*

The financials above are impressive enough, even though illustrative, for investors to take a serious look at this line of business, for this is surely going to play a significant part in the healthcare monitoring and delivery services in the months and years ahead.

---

[6] http://www.prb.org/Publications/Reports/2012/india-older-population.aspx

Table 10.4 Pro forma I & E example for remote care

Remote care						
All figures ₹ 000's	Year 0	Year 1	Year 2	Year 3	Year 4	Year 5
Total number of subscribers at the end of the applicable year		1200	2400	3600	4800	6000
Charges (per month)		3	3.3	3.63	3.99	4.39
Remote care personnel salary, room rent, power, connectivity and cloud hosting costs		(14,475)	(15,923)	(17,515)	(19,266)	(21,193)
Clinician (non-clinician) salary		(20)	(22)	(24)	(27)	(29)
Total clinician payment		(15600)	(48,840)	(88,572)	(1,35,762)	(1,91,504)
I & E statement						
Income	0	23,400	73,260	1,32,858	2,03,643	2,87,256
Loans (for capital expenditures)	(51000)	0	0	0	0	0
COGS	0	(35,175)	(69,863)	(1,11,187)	(1,60,128)	(2,17,797)
Depreciation	0	(10,200)	(10,200)	(10,200)	(10,200)	(10,200)
EBIT	0	(21,975)	(6803)	11,471	33,315	59,259
Interest costs	0	(4561)	(3613)	(2471)	(1105)	516
Payable IT	0	0	0	(2970)	(10,629)	(19,726)
EAT	0	(26,536)	(10,415)	6030	21,580	40,050
Free cash flow	(51000)	(16,336)	(215)	16,230	31,780	50,250
NPV @ 6.25%	8482					
IRR	10%					

Change Management

[*Much of the following material is based on the basic principles of clinical transformation as propounded by Perot Systems and promoted by HIMSS.*[7]]

The Greek philosopher Heraclitus believed that perpetual change is the natural law by which the universe operates.[8] He never claimed that change would be pleasant or that anyone would be eager to embrace it. In fact, change is inherently stressful, a precarious balance between harmony and discord between what's comfortable and what's risky. Heraclitus' perspectives on change, formulated 2500 years ago, uncannily presage the efforts of today's business enterprises to respond to the challenges of changing their business models and relationships.

---

[7] Health Information and Management Systems Society
[8] http://mthink.com/legacy/www.hctproject.com/content/white_papers/HCT1_wp_friedman.htm

Healthcare providers are especially aware of the need to implement key changes in the way healthcare is delivered, to provide safer, more cost-effective care to their patients. They have also learned, occasionally through painful experiences, that a purely technical solution — putting laptops in every hospital room, for example — does little to improve the quality and safety of patient care.[9]

The readers will do well to note that whenever telemedicine is introduced, there will be an inevitable impact on the various business processes running at that time. The impact levels can be from minimal to totally disruptive. So, change management assumes enormous importance. For this, the first step is to perform a business impact analysis followed by a business process re-engineering.

Any change management requires paying attention to people, process and technology in equal degrees. Just concentrating on technology is a major mistake and has led to IT implementation failures in healthcare far too frequently for anybody's comfort. Recognising the need to handle the technological aspects is easy. The need to handle people and processes is not much.

From both organisational and people perspective, any change is a significant disruption. The hitherto usual way of working is supplanted by an entirely new way. The good part about telemedicine is that the impact of its introduction is varied. Where only teleconsultations are being done from a specially dedicated room, the effect is minimal. When the full range of telemonitoring is introduced in both the wards and individual rooms, the effect is maximal.

It is wiser to get the people whose way of working is going to be impacted fully on board from day 1. Ramming it down the throat by presenting it as some sort of a *fait accompli* is a very bad idea and should never be done – it almost guarantees hostility and usually results in total failure making it a non-starter from very first day of the project.

Incidentally, the most sceptical people usually turn out to be the most ardent supporters once their fears are allayed, and concerns are addressed satisfactorily. Regular training, letting them help set up the equipment and using for practice runs are all great methods to not only prepare them for the upcoming change but also make them comfortable using the various instruments in a less stressful manner.

Necessary changes in the existing processes need to be taken care of too. The existing processes will need careful evaluation as they will need to undergo none to minimal to maximal changes. Some may need to be entirely scrapped while introducing new ones. Depending on the amount of changes, investing in a qualified change management expert with proven track record will turn out to be a wise choice.

Certain guiding principles to manage the overall change are as follows:

- Reframing the organisational culture
- Creating improvement capability
- Collaborating across teams
- Taking evidence-based decisions
- Driving results and benefits
- Maintaining constancy and ongoing focus
- Allocating resources appropriately and wisely

---

[9] mthink.com/legacy/www.hctproject.com/content/white_papers/HCT1_wp_friedman.htm

Diffusion of Innovation[10]

The application of telemedicine technology as a whole is not really innovative anymore. Neither is teleconsultation nor telepresence nor robotics. Telemonitoring and remote care, perhaps. Yet, it has largely not been as common place as it ought to have. This is somewhat bewildering. Therefore, it is worthwhile to try and understand the reasons for the things having to come to such a pass.

The answer is multifactorial – not the right solution for a given situation, pricing not right, things not going according to plan, people not convinced of its effectiveness, etc. The list is large.

Perhaps the most important reason is the lack of conviction amongst the stakeholders in terms of doctors, nurses, patients and payers that this technology actually makes a difference. This could be a consequence of not having or using the most appropriate solution for a particular situation.

Not everyone will benefit from teleconsultation using telepresence and far-end camera control – it is neither necessary nor indeed does it work in every encounter. Robotic surgery is not necessary for every surgical procedure. Therefore, some other innovative telemedicine technology solutions are required to be used to help address the various healthcare delivery-related issues of the day.

The challenge that continues to remain is in ensuring the success of these innovations in terms of widespread acceptance and use. For this, it is important to try and understand as to how the various stakeholders can be convinced to join the bandwagon in large numbers. The answer lies in knowing how any innovation becomes popular.

In his "Diffusion of Innovations" in 1995, Everett Rogers argued that "diffusion is the process by which an innovation is communicated through certain channels over time among the members of a social system".[11]

Innovation is defined as "an idea, practice, or object that is perceived to be new by an individual or other unit of adoption".

Communication is defined as "a process by which participants create and share information with one another to reach a mutual understanding".

The phrase "Diffusion of innovation" itself is defined as "the process by which an innovation is communicated over a period of time among the members of a social system".

Rogers states that the innovation itself occurs in four stages as under:

1. Invention
2. Diffusion (or communication) through the social system
3. Time
4. Consequences

---

[10] www.peecworks.org/PEEC/PEEC_Gen/I01795F8D; www.d.umn.edu/~lrochfor/ireland/dif-of-in-ch06.pdf

[11] web.stanford.edu/class/symbsys205/Diffusion%20of%20Innovations.htm

The original diffusion research was done as early as 1903 by the French sociologist Gabriel Tarde. Subsequently in the 1940s, two sociologists, Bryce Ryan and Neal Gross, published their seminal study of the diffusion of hybrid seed among Iowa farmers where they classified the adopter categories as under (their corresponding population-distribution rates are provided alongside) (Table 10.5).

Ryan and Gross found that one of the most important characteristics of the innovators, apart from the fact that they were of higher socioeconomic status than later adopters, is that they required a shorter adoption period than any other category.

Rogers additionally identified several additional characteristics dominant in the various innovation adopter types as follows (Table 10.6).

Rogers breaks the process of adoption of innovation itself broadly down into five stages as follows (Table 10.7).

Table 10.5 Adopter category with distribution rate

S. no.	Adopter category	Population distribution (%)
1	Innovators	2.5
2	Early adopters	13.5
3	Early majority	34
4	Late majority	34
5	Laggards	16

Table 10.6 Adopter characteristics

Adopter category	Characteristics
Innovator	They are venturesome, desire for the rash, the daring and the risky and have control of substantial financial resources that enable them to absorb possible loss from an unprofitable innovation. They also have the ability to understand and apply complex technical knowledge and possess the ability to cope with a high degree of uncertainty associated with an innovation
Early adopters	Aka "opinion leaders", they are an integrated part of the local social system having the greatest degree of opinion leadership in most systems, serve as role models for other members or the society, are respected by peers for their judicious, well-informed decision-making and are successful people
Early majority	Constituting one-third of the members of a system, they interact frequently with peers seldom holding positions of opinion leadership themselves and mostly deliberate long and hard before adopting a new idea and not going by a mere "hunch"
Late majority	Also constitute one-third of the members of a system who adopt due to pressure from peers and economic necessity and are generally sceptical as well as cautious
Laggard	The constituents of this group possess no opinion leadership, are isolates, have their point of reference in the past, are suspicious of innovations, whose innovation-decision process is lengthy, and have limited resources

Table 10.7 Adoption stages

S. no.	Adoption stage	Description
1	Awareness	The individual is exposed to the innovation but lacks complete information about it
2	Interest	The individual becomes interested in the new idea and seeks additional information about it
3	Evaluation	The individual mentally applies the innovation to his present and anticipated future situation and then decides whether or not to try it
4	Trial	The individual makes full use of the innovation
5	Adoption	The individual decides to continue with the full use of the innovation

When the decisions to adopt are neither authoritative nor collective, each member of the social system faces his own innovation-decision that too follows a five-step process as below:

1. **Knowledge**: the person becomes aware of an innovation and has some idea of how it functions.
2. **Persuasion**: the person forms a favourable, or an unfavourable, attitude towards innovation.
3. **Decision**: the person engages in activities that lead to a choice being adopted or rejected.
4. **Implementation**: the person puts an innovation to use.
5. **Confirmation**: the person evaluates the results of an innovation-decision already made.

Rogers states that people will adopt an innovation if they believe that it will ultimately enhance their utility. They must therefore believe that the innovation is most likely to yield some advantage relative to the idea it aims to supersede. Therefore, the challenge for any innovation to succeed is to convince the key opinion leaders, who are to be found amongst the early adopters, of its overall usefulness. A critical momentum is gained once the early majority use it and get some amongst the late majority to adopt it too. Laggards will however always be there. It is wise to accept and tolerate it irrespective of how galling it is.

Another important point to note is that the most hostile elements turn out to be the biggest champions once successfully convinced. So, concentrating on them early on and convincing them is well worth the effort. No one evangelises better than a converted heretic.

Legal Aspects

11

Abstract

This chapter discusses, in brief, the various legal issues involved with respect to telemedicine services.

Overview

Legal problems are always an ultrasensitive issue, more so because most of the stakeholders generally remain oblivious, to varying degrees, of all the applicable laws and how best to handle them.

The best way to mitigate this in healthcare context is to have a legally valid and safe informed consent or similar contract executed before the fact, i.e. before rendering services. This is true for telemedicine services too.

Definitions

Privacy is ensuring that private information indeed remains private and that no one is able to gain access without permission from the owner of the information in any context that is crucial.

Confidentiality is keeping or causing things to be kept secret or private.

Secrecy is ensuring that secrets are kept and no one can learn anything about them.

Security is ensuring that no one, known or unknown, is able to "steal" information.

Consent is providing permission for agreement to do something or allowing something to take place.

© Springer Nature Singapore Pte Ltd. 2017   107
S.B. Bhattacharyya, *A DIY Guide to Telemedicine for Clinicians*,
DOI 10.1007/978-981-10-5305-4_11

Informed consent, in healthcare context, is a process to get permission from a person for conducting a healthcare intervention on him. It must always be taken before initiating the event.

Indemnification is an agreement executed between two parties that provide for one party to bear the monetary costs, either directly or by reimbursement, for losses incurred by the other party, usually as a consequence of legal action.

Medical Records Legal Status

In case of medical records, the person whose details are gathered is the patient who is the owner of his records and all of its contents (since it contains information about him), while the ones who actually create the records are the care providers (to whom the information has been conveyed in confidence to ensure that the right care is delivered).

The onus therefore is on the providers to act as the custodian of all such records and hold its contents on behalf of the owner as a matter of trust at all times taking due and proper care to ensure that these are not divulged to any third party without explicit consent from the owner who has expressed his consent on being duly informed about his rights and privileges with respect to the record and its contents.

Licence to Practice Issues

These are restricted geography-wise—not everyone can practice healthcare anywhere and everywhere. Needless to say, this makes practicing telemedicine a tricky matter as by its very nature the various services are delivered in the cyberspace without any consideration to the actual physical location of either the provider or the receiver.

The author's take on this, provided without prejudice, is as follows:

1. If the encounter is that of teleconsultation and the patient is physically located in a geography where the clinician is not licensed to practise, he should not provide any consultation to the patient and instead should insist that a clinician, who has the necessary licence, discuss the case with him and provide the actual care undertaking all the legal liabilities as the primary physician. It is additionally preferable that this clinician be physically present with the receiver for the entire duration of the teleconsultation.
2. If the encounter is of telereferral, then the clinician requesting the referral is the primary physician and assumes all legal responsibilities that arise.
3. If the encounter is telemonitoring and the clinician travels to a geography where he is not licensed to practise, then a peculiar situation arises since the patient continues to be physically located where the clinician is legally licensed to practise while the clinician is not. In such situations the clinician may be "deemed" to be in the same geography as the patient and may thus conduct telemonitoring sessions. *It is to be noted here that in such situations the author considers that the patient's location determines the licensing privileges and not the clinician's*

location. Under these circumstances, the clinician should be able to provide services without falling foul of the law. Needless to say, this matter is contentious and is open to legal challenges. Hence, due caution should be adopted when providing care in this particular scenario.

4. For remote care, which is basically an advanced form of telemonitoring, there should ideally be no problem since no care is actually provided and only some further actions are undertaken as follows. When any anomaly/problem is noted, the fact is noted and either someone is physically sent to the receiver for further evaluation and action or the receiver is asked to physically visit some facility or clinician (or provider). *It is advisable that the entity providing remote care services (telehomecare and remote monitoring) take appropriate legal defence in form of end-user consent, indemnification of the stakeholders, etc., to ensure that the laws of the land where the person being monitored physically resides is strictly adhered to at all times. Since the remote care monitoring servers are located in the Cloud and the monitoring by persons can be done from anywhere (as long as they are in the cyberspace), the physical location of the person (or patient) is the determinant factor for all matters legal.*

Special Considerations

Telemedicine services, like any other line of business, are essentially a contract between the care provider (clinician) and the care receiver (patient) where the care provider promises to deliver a set of previously agreed upon services, expressed explicitly or implicitly, to the care receiver for a previously agreed upon fee that the latter promises to pay to the former.

Disputes arise when either party, or both, feel aggrieved about the non-fulfilment of the terms of the contract by the other party, as per their assessment. As long as both the parties are able to resolve their differences through mutual discussions or arbitration to the satisfaction of the aggrieved party, things work rather well. In those cases where such measures fail, there is no alternative to litigating in order to seek redressal from the competent courts of law.

Needless to say, the lesser the opportunity for negative assessments of any nature, the greater the satisfaction levels achieved by the various stakeholders with respect to telemedicine.

Concluding Remarks

When in doubt, ask, especially where law is involved.

Legal entanglements should be avoided to the maximal possible extent even in the best of times. This does not however mean that one should permit oneself to be paralysed by fear. One must not be risk averse but not reckless either—that should be the dictum to be followed.

Conclusion

That day is not far away when much of the health-related encounters will be conducted "virtually" using telemedicine technology, ultimately culminating in a situation where this mode is the one of choice rather than of exception.

Telemedicine is an exciting technology and continues to hold the promise of being truly transformational in terms of healthcare delivery to everyone's benefit. As the population continues to grow at a rate faster than the concomitant growth in the number of available qualified clinicians and facilities (institutional beds, investigation laboratories, day-care centres, etc.), this technology will need to be optimally harnessed to ensure that all those who need care are catered to at least at acceptable levels, if not the best possible.

As more persons are cared for without them having to crowd the institutions, the care providers will be able to "visit" the patients under their care anytime from anywhere without having to physically travel, and those requiring continuous monitoring cared for with proactive interventions, it will definitely lead to a situation where only those who actually need to have a physical encounter with their clinicians will need to travel and be attended to. This will help address many of the issues that currently challenge the system. The patient load in the facilities will come down, and clinicians will need to travel less and be able to devote more time and effort on those patients who actually need such attention.

Telemedicine will definitely improve both communication and levels of satisfaction. Although costs and their reimbursements coupled with legal aspects will continue to remain a factor, the increased use of the technology will usher in a greater degree of confidence in it allowing all stakeholders to learn the optimal ways and means of harnessing the technology, which will in turn ease the underlying pressures that continue to limit its widespread use.

Transforming anything is not easy. Changing the old order and ushering in the new are both hard and painful, a process that is bound to be met with resistance to varying degrees at least in the beginning. However, not keeping things "fresh" is most unwise. Things become "stale" when the rot sets in and before long it's all

© Springer Nature Singapore Pte Ltd. 2017   111
S.B. Bhattacharyya, *A DIY Guide to Telemedicine for Clinicians*,
DOI 10.1007/978-981-10-5305-4

moribund, which is not at all desirable at any time. Consequently, innovation is a must. Yet for it to become a commonplace, a long gestation period is required. This is particularly so in healthcare where severely entrenched ideas and the ways of doing things are jealously guarded and aggressively defended.

There are however many ways to skin this particular cat. By following sound scientific methods that are backed up by proven management processes, it is possible to ensure satisfactory outcomes. Telemedicine is not only important but necessary in order to make the required "course correction" to the care delivery processes. The informed patient armed with easy accessibility to the latest "buzz" is not only wiser but also anxious due to the many points of view propounded by the many "experts" who infest the media jungle of the modern day and age out there. To best "guide" and ensure that he is able to get proper care, it has become imperative to properly harness the currently available tools to optimal extents.

The author truly hopes that this DIY Guide will help clinicians to not only be in step with the times but also make a real difference to their patients as well as in the way they collaborate to deliver even better care on a continual basis. The various information and steps necessary to set up and run a telemedicine service have been provided in these pages before. However, the author expects the readers to use these information to act as a trigger for them to help plan the services that are right for their practice.

Telemedicine Practice Home Truths

Some Dos and Don'ts:

1. *Premium non nocere* [Lat.] – firstly, do no harm.
2. An unwell person cannot be expected to be in his "right" frame of mind; the more critical a patient is, the more anxious his relations and attendants will be; and consequently they will need to be handled with the greatest degrees of sensitivity and understanding.
3. The prevailing laws of the location where the care services are delivering from and that of the location where the patient is located at the time of receiving the delivered care must be noted and obeyed at all times without exception.
4. With respect to India, it is necessary to carefully note that the prevailing Indian cyber laws provide unlimited liabilities and prison terms of up to 10 years demanding that due care be taken at all times when using digital health systems.
5. One must always respect patient's rights to privacy, confidentiality and ownership of their data.
6. One must never forget that as a clinician one is the sacred guardian of the patient's data till eternity.
7. One must conduct proper due diligence before offering or not a particular service or a group thereof – it is always wiser to be proactive instead of reactive.
8. Without access to a patient's relevant past records, EMR/EHR, it is most unwise to perform any type of consultation, including telemedicine, anytime – in fact, it should not be done at all.
9. Every record needs to be authenticated, either through digital signatures or non-repudiable observer identification with date and time stamping, to be legally valid.
10. Audit log of every action, without exception, must be maintained at all times.
11. Simplest solutions are usually the best one in most cases.
12. One must never overlook connectivity and power supply issues.
13. Telemonitoring can be automated, but every anticipated output needs to be validated by a human with appropriate levels of authorisation to make it legally valid.
14. Monitoring, especially in chronic illnesses, follow-up reviews, referral consultations, etc., are better suited for telemedicine instead of initial evaluation.

© Springer Nature Singapore Pte Ltd. 2017
S.B. Bhattacharyya, *A DIY Guide to Telemedicine for Clinicians*,
DOI 10.1007/978-981-10-5305-4

15. Telemedicine is best for triage rather than treatment in cases of emergency or out-of-hours consultations.
16. Telemedicine must not be used to completely replace the need for any physical interaction between the patient and provider; the world is not ready yet for that.
17. It is both important and necessary to recognise that the patients need to be able to communicate with their clinicians whenever they want to irrespective of where each other might be; it is increasingly becoming more of a need than a want as time goes by.
18. Telemedicine ought to be treated as a cost centre that produces revenues indirectly (as opposed to profit centres that produce revenues directly). Consequently, both prudence and discipline are required to ensure that the costs do not gallop out of control.
19. Pricing must always be fair and not even appear to be fleecing –while every business exists to make profits, profit-taking itself needs to be tempered to ensure that it does not become to be seen as profiteering.
20. Patient consent must be taken before beginning of the session, preferably each time – a one-time blanket consent is open to criticism and being concluded to be bad in law.

Glossary

2G/3G/4G The "generation" of the underlying wireless network technology.

ADSL Asymmetric digital subscriber line (ADSL) is a type of digital subscriber line (DSL) broadband communications technology used for connecting to the Internet. ADSL allows more data at high speeds to be sent over existing copper telephone lines (POTS – plain old telephone system), when compared to traditional modem lines.

AMC Annual maintenance contract.

Biosensor A device which uses a living organism or biological molecules, especially enzymes or antibodies, to detect the presence of chemicals.

Bluetooth® Bluetooth is a wireless technology standard for exchanging data over short distances (using short-wavelength UHF radio waves in the ISM band from 2.4 to 2.485 GHz) from fixed and mobile devices to building personal area networks (PANs). A Bluetooth® device uses radio waves instead of wires or cables to connect to a phone or computer. When two Bluetooth devices want to talk to each other, they need to pair. *It however is not safe from hacking as many think it to be.*

Breakeven Point The exact point where total income equals total expenditure. Over and above this point, all earnings are pure profits.

CDMA/GSM CDMA (Code Division Multiple Access) and GSM (Global System for Mobiles) are shorthand for the two major radio systems used in cell phones. Both acronyms tend to be grouped together as a bunch of technologies run by the same entities.

Clinician The provider of the healthcare services. Can be individual like the clinical staff, doctor, dentist, nursing staff, paramedical staff, physiotherapist, podiatrist, healthcare worker, etc., as well as institutional like hospital, nursing home, hospice, day-care facility, clinic, doctor's chamber, polyclinic, etc.

Cloud Computing The practice of using a network of remote servers hosted on the Internet to store, manage and process data, rather than a local server or a personal computer.

Continua Health Alliance Continua Health Alliance is an international non-profit, open industry group of nearly 240 healthcare providers, communications, medical and fitness device companies. Personal Connected Health Alliance members

© Springer Nature Singapore Pte Ltd. 2017
S.B. Bhattacharyya, *A DIY Guide to Telemedicine for Clinicians*,
DOI 10.1007/978-981-10-5305-4

aim to develop a system to deliver personal and individual healthcare. Continua was a founding member of Personal Connected Health Alliance which was launched in February 2014 with other founding members mHealth SUMMIT and HIMSS.

Cost Driver The unit of an activity that causes the change in activity's cost, i.e. drives the cost one way or the other.

CPOE Acronym for computerised physician order entry. Some substitute provider for physician since many orders are actually posted by a nursing staff or paramedic. However, the ultimate legal responsibility lies with the primary care physician. These systems are used to post-treatment-related orders that are investigation related (both laboratory and radiodiagnostics); disease management related like medications, procedures (including surgical procedures), diet and lifestyle; or administrative related like referral, admission, discharge, transfer, follow-up, etc.

DICOM DICOM is acronym of Digital Imaging and Communication and is an image format with special characteristics. These images permit users to change contrasts, annotate (these can be personalised per user), enlarged, miniaturised area and volume measurements calculated, etc. They do however need specialised viewers for proper screen rendering, manipulation and annotation.

EHR Electronic health record is a longitudinal electronic record providing information about the health of an individual composed by serially arranging in ascending order by date and time from the very first EMR to the most recent of the individual, essentially a health dashboard that permits providers to get an overall view of the health status of the person including progress and maintenance thereof at a glance.

EMR Electronic medical record is the record of a single provider-receiver medical encounter in any care setting – outpatients, inpatients, accident and emergency or home care; there can be several EMRs generated during one episode or one admission.

Encounter A clinical encounter is defined by ASTM as "(1) an instance of direct provider/practitioner to patient interaction, regardless of the setting, between a patient and a practitioner vested with primary responsibility for diagnosing, evaluating or treating the patient's condition, or both, or providing social worker services. (2) A contact between a patient and a practitioner who has primary responsibility for assessing and treating the patient at a given contact, exercising independent judgment". Encounter serves as a focal point linking clinical, administrative and financial information and occur in many different settings – ambulatory care, inpatient care, emergency care, home healthcare and field and virtual (telemedicine).

Episode An episode of care consists of all clinically related services for one patient for a discrete diagnostic condition from the onset of symptoms until the treatment is complete (http://www.ncmedsoc.org/non_members/pai/PAI-FinalWorkbookforVideo.pdf). Thus, for every new problem or set of problems that a person visits his clinical clinician is considered a new episode. Within that episode the patient will have one or many encounters with his clinical clinicians till the treatment for that episode is complete. Even before the resolution of an episode, the person may have a new episode that is considered as a distinctly separate event altogether. Thus, there may be none, one or several ongoing active episodes. All resolved episodes are considered inactive and are thus considered as part of the patient's past history. A notable point here is that all chronic diseases are considered active and may never get resolved during the lifetime of the person, e.g. diabetes mellitus, hypertension, etc.

Expected Volume This is same as current volumes and growing at a particular rate per year.

FV This is the value of an asset on a specific date and measures the nominal future sum of money that a given sum of money is "worth" at a specified time in the future assuming a certain interest rate or, more generally, rate of return. This index is helpful in figuring out the likely effects of investments to have in the future of the business, all things remaining exactly as they are as on date.

GPRS General Packet Radio Service is a packet-oriented mobile data service on the 2G and 3G cellular communication system's global system for mobile communications (GSM).

Growth Factor This represents the growth rate of anything, not just profits or sales. However, normally this term is applied to annual growth in business. Naturally, a positive growth factor represents a growing business while a negative growth factor represents a shrinking one.

Hadoop Hadoop is an open source, Java-based programming framework that supports the processing and storage of extremely large data sets in a distributed computing environment. It is part of the Apache project sponsored by the Apache Software Foundation. It's core parts are Hadoop Distributed File System (HDFS), which is a virtual file system that looks like any other file system except that whenever any file is moved on to HDFS, it is split into many small files and each of those files are replicated and stored on several servers (usually three) for fault tolerance constraints, and Hadoop MapReduce, which is a way to split every request into smaller bits that are then sent to many small servers for processing with the results then combined back to convey the appearance of a single action, allowing a truly scalable use of CPU power.

Health The World Health Organization (WHO) defines health as "a state of complete physical, mental and social well-being and not merely the absence of disease or infirmity" (1948 constitution).

Home Care Care delivered in the home of the patient.

IoT Internet of things is the interconnection via the Internet of computing devices embedded in everyday objects, enabling them to send and receive data.

IRR Internal rate of return is the interest rate at which the net present value of all the cash flows (both positive and negative) from a project or investment equal zero and is used to evaluate the attractiveness of a project or investment – usually, the higher the better.

ISDN Integrated Services Digital Network (ISDN) was first defined in 1988 and is a set of communication standards for simultaneous digital transmission of voice, video, data and other network services over the traditional circuits of the public switched telephone network. Although still available and used for dedicated videoconferencing, most of its functionalities are now handled using either dedicated fibre-optic cabling network (less common) or ADSL (more common).

LIS Acronym for laboratory information system. Such systems ideally track a sample from the point of its collection to its eventual reporting. Users (pathologists, biochemists, microbiologists, virologists, serologists, etc.) are not only able to track samples and report them but also manage a rigorous quality control process using such systems. They are usually interfaced with semi-auto and autoanalysers so that sample reporting can also be automated, permitting the processing and reporting of a large number of samples easy.

MAR Acronym for Medical Administration Record (system). This is also known by its other name medication reconciliation. These systems help track the administration of various medications prescribed for a patient and the various issues involved in that process like date and time of administration, adverse reactions, reasons for patient refusal, nonadministration of a medication or dose thereof, etc.

mHealth mHealth (mobile health) is a general term for the use of mobile phones and other wireless technology in medical care. The most common application of mHealth is the use of mobile phones and communication devices to educate consumers about preventive healthcare services.

MLLN Managed leased line network (MLLN) is a system that can provide leased line connectivity, that is, a dedicated telecommunication path between two fixed points.

NFC Near-field communication (NFC) is a short-range wireless connectivity standard (Ecma-340, ISO/IEC 18092) that uses magnetic field induction to enable communication between devices to establish communication by bringing them within 4 cm (1.6 in.) of each other.

NIM Acronym for nursing information module. These information management systems deal with matters related to nursing and managing nursing care delivery like nursing care records, care evaluation, discharge planning, workload assessment, resource management, etc.

NPV Net present value is the difference between the present value of cash inflows and the present value of cash outflows and is used in capital budgeting to analyse the profitability of a projected investment or project – usually, the higher the better.

OEM Original equipment manufacturer is an entity that manufactures a part or subsystem that is used in another entity's end product.

PACS PACS is acronym for picture archival and communication system. This basically is the storage system specially designed for storing radiodiagnostic images. Using an RIS along with PACS ensures that the images can be easily accessed, viewed, annotated and sent to wherever these are needed. It must be noted here that a RIS and a PACS are not interdependent but are mutually exclusive instead. Either can function on their own. In fact, most radiodiagnostic devices come with their own inbuilt PACS systems. However, if a corresponding RIS is connected to these PACS, the RIS can manage DICOM images in several PACS and help provide an integrated view of all images from a single patient, making a radiodiagnostician/physician review of the patient all that more comprehensive.

Patient The receiver of the healthcare services, usually the patient.

PDA Personal digital assistant is a palmtop computer that is programmable and functions as a personal organiser but also provides email and Internet access.

Predatory Pricing The pricing of goods or services at such a low level that other firms cannot compete and are forced to leave the market.

Preventive Care Preventive healthcare (alternately preventive medicine or prophylaxis) consists of measures taken for disease prevention, as opposed to disease treatment. Health, disease and disability are dynamic processes which begin before individuals realise they are affected.

Pricing Price is the value that is put to a product or service and is the result of a complex set of calculations, research and understanding and risk-taking ability.

Pricing Strategy Strategy for determining pricing of products and/or services and takes into account segments, ability to pay, market conditions, competitor actions, trade margins and input costs, amongst others and is targeted at the defined customers and against competitors.

Privacy Freedom from damaging publicity, public scrutiny, secret surveillance or unauthorized disclosure of one's personal data or information, as by a government, corporation or individual.

PV Present value is the current worth of a future sum of money or stream of cash flows given a specified rate of return. Future cash flows are discounted at the discount rate (usually market rate or WACC). The higher the rate, the lower the present value of the future cash flows.

RFID Radio frequency identification is a technology that incorporates the use of electromagnetic or electrostatic coupling in the radio frequency (RF) portion of the electromagnetic spectrum to uniquely identify an object, animal or person.

RIS Acronym for radiology (or radiodiagnostic) information system. These systems provide a composite interface to manage the images, especially for reporting. Most radiodiagnostic devices have the necessary digital image generation, capture and storing functionalities apart from using the devices themselves like positioning the patient, moving the gantry, etc.

Secrecy The action of keeping something secret or the state of being kept secret.

SaaD Software as a drug, aka digital therapeutics, deploys software modules as an enhancement, or even as a substitute, to a drug and is used in chronic conditions where it combines the latest developments in terms of behavioural economics, smartphones, gamification, biometric sensors, data analytics and machine learning to pre-emptively try and improve health outcomes.

Satellite Communication satellites act by bouncing signals received from a sending (or uploading) dish located somewhere to a receiving dish somewhere else, suitably boosting them in the process, acting somewhat like a giant mirror cum signal booster in space. Orbiting geostationary satellites located 22,300 miles above the Earth's equator and having the ability to receive and transmit data using a relatively small satellite dish on Earth called VSAT (Very Small Aperture Terminal), which is a satellite communications system that serves home and business users. The end user needs a box that interfaces between the user's computer and an outside antenna with a transceiver (capable of both transmitting and receiving). The transceiver receives or sends a signal to a satellite transponder in the sky. The satellite sends and receives signals from an Earth station computer that acts as a hub for the system. Each end user is interconnected with the hub station via the satellite in a star topology. For one end user to communicate with another, each transmission has to first go from his transceiver to a hub station that then retransmits the signal via the satellite to the other end user's VSAT transceiver dish. The communication system is capable of handling data, voice and video signals and is the satellite communication technology most widely used to provide telemedicine services.

Sunk Cost A cost that has been incurred and is not expected to/cannot be recovered.

SVA Shareholder value added is expressed as a company's capital costs from stock and bond issues subtracted from its earnings after tax (EAT).

Telemetry The process of recording and transmitting the readings of an instrument.

Telepresence The use of virtual reality technology to create a sensation of being somewhere other than their actual location.

WACC Weighted average cost of capital is the average rate of return a company expects to incur as borrowing costs of capital and is expected to pay as interest to its creditors (investors). As a "thumb rule", this is 1.5 times the prevailing inflation rate. However, should the prevailing market interest rate be higher, then that figure has to be considered.

Wellness Wellness is the optimal state of health of individuals and groups. There are two focal concerns: realisation of the fullest potential of an individual physically, psychologically, socially, spiritually and economically and the fulfilment of one's role expectations in the family, community, place of worship, workplace and other settings.

Wi-Fi This is a popular but trademarked phrase that represents a catchier name for IEEE 802.11b direct sequence and means IEEE 802.11× communication protocol and has an associated logo (refer to the ecosystem figures provided in the later chapters). Incidentally, Wi-Fi was chosen from a list that included Trapeze, Skybridge, Hornet and Dragonfly and is a wireless networking technology that uses radio waves to provide wireless high-speed Internet and network connections.

WiMAX Worldwide Interoperability for Microwave Access is a family of wireless communication standards based on the IEEE 802.16 set of standards that provide multiple physical layer (PHY) and media access control (MAC) options.

ZigBee This is an open global standard for wireless technology designed to use low-power digital radio signals for personal area networks. It operates on the IEEE 802.15.4 specification and is used to create networks that require a low data transfer rate, energy efficiency and secure networking.

References

1. Adapted from "Recommendations On Guidelines, Standards & Practices For Telemedicine In India", Version 1.0, July 2006, Recommendations of National Taskforce on Telemedicine, constituted by an order of Ministry of Health & Family Welfare, Government of India.
2. Carroll R et al. IEEE pervasive computing magazine, continua: an interoperable personal healthcare ecosystem, Oct–Dec 2007.
3. searchmobilecomputing.techtarget.com/definition/.
4. www.investopedia.com/terms/.
5. www.explainthatstuff.com/.
6. www.groundcontrol.com/How_Does_Satellite_Internet_Work.htm.
7. searchnetworking.techtarget.com/definition/satellite-Internet-connection.
8. ccm.net/faq/2761-what-is-network-architecture.
9. www.profitableventure.com.
10. cchpca.org.
11. The internet of things for medical devices—Prospects, challenges and the way forward; Ashok Khanna, Prateep Mishra; TCS White Paper.
12. Medical internet of things and big data in healthcare; Dimiter V. Dimitrov, MD, PhD; Diavita Ltd., Varna, Bulgaria.
13. Applying Research Evidence to Optimize Telehomecare; Kathryn H. Bowles, PhD, RN and Amy C. Baugh, MSN, RN. https://www.ncbi.nlm.nih.gov/pmc/articles/PMC2874189/.
14. en.wikipedia.org.
15. searchhealthit.techtarget.com/definition/.
16. Friedman D. Change management: an integral component of clinical transformation. HCT Project—A thought leadership project from Montgomery Research, Inc.
17. internetofthingsagenda.techtarget.com.
18. connectedhealth.partners.org/about/what-is-connected-health/default.aspx.
19. www.studytonight.com/computer-networks/network-topology-types.
20. Toromanovic S, Hasanovic E, Masic I. Nursing information systems. Mater Sociomed. 2010;22(3):168–71. www.ncbi.nlm.nih.gov/pmc/articles/PMC3813545/.
21. The Difference Between a Business Case and a Business Plan By Gabriel Steinhardt.
22. www.marketwired.com/press-release/psilos-group-digital-therapeutics-software-as-drug-is-6-billion-potential-market-opportunity-2164437.htm.
23. www1.lsbu.ac.uk/water/enztech/biosensors.html.
24. Biosensors By A. Pooja Shukla, SRM University. www.slideshare.net/951384/biosensors-33317356.
25. HEALTH MONITORING SYSTEM, K.L.Nishitha, R. Ravi Kumar; Department of ECE, KL University, Vaddeswaram, Guntur, Andhra Pradesh, India. www.ijirset.com/upload/may/13_%20HEALTH.pdf.
26. A Hospital Healthcare Monitoring System Using Wireless Sensor Networks; Media Aminian and Hamid Reza Naji; Iran. www.omicsonline.org/a-hospital-healthcare-monitoring-system-using-wireless-sensor-networks-2157-7420.1000121.php?aid=11778.
27. cecs.wright.edu/cart/wearable-portable%20health%20monitoring%20system.html.

© Springer Nature Singapore Pte Ltd. 2017
S.B. Bhattacharyya, *A DIY Guide to Telemedicine for Clinicians*,
DOI 10.1007/978-981-10-5305-4

28. Health Monitoring and Management Using Internet-of-Things (IoT) Sensing with Cloud-based Processing: Opportunities and Challenges; Moeen Hassanalieragh, Alex Page, Tolga Soyata, Gaurav Sharma, Mehmet Aktas, Gonzalo Mateos, Burak Kantarci, Silvana Andreescu; USA. www.ece.rochester.edu/~gsharma/papers/Moeen_HealthMonitor_SCC2015.pdf.

29. PATIENT HEALTH MONITORING SYSTEM (PHMS) USING IoT DEVICES; Aruna Devi. S, Godfrey Winster. S, Sasikumar. S; Department of Computer Science and Engineering, Saveetha Engineering College, Chennai, India. www.ijcset.com/docs/IJCSET16-07-03-039.pdf.

30. Secured Smart Healthcare Monitoring System Based on Iot; Bhoomika. B.K, Dr. K N Muralidhara; PES college of Engineering, Mandya. www.ijritcc.org/download/1438757194.pdf.

31. Secured Smart Healthcare Monitoring System Based on IOT; Duddela Dileep Kumar, Pratti Venkateswarlu. www.imperialjournals.com/index.php/IJIR/article/view/2325.

32. Smart Health Care System Using Internet of Things; K. Natarajan, B. Prasath, P. Kokila; Nandha Engineering College, Erode, Tamil Nadu, India. www.jncet.org/Manuscripts/Volume-6/Issue-3/Vol-6-issue-3-M-10.pdf.

33. Highly Secured IoT Based Health Care System for Elderly People using Body Sensor Network; Snehal Sanjay Kale, D. S. Bhagwat; Department of E&TC, Indira College of Engineering and Management, Pune, Maharashtra, India. www.ijirset.com/upload/2016/october/42_SNEHAL_KALE_IJIRSET_PAPER%20_1_.pdf.

34. Patient Health Monitoring System using IoT and Android; Meria M George, Nimmy Mary Cyriac, Sobin Mathew, Tess Antony; Department of Information Technology Department of Information Technology, Amal Jyothi College of Engineering, MG University, Amal Jyothi College of Engineering, MG University, Kottayam, Kerala, India. www.journal4research.org/articles/J4RV2I1036.pdf.

35. www.hindawi.com/journals/bmri/2012/546021/.

36. scholarworks.wmich.edu/cgi/viewcontent.cgi?article=1661&context=masters_theses.

37. managedhealthcareexecutive.modernmedicine.com/mhe/Technology/Clinical-transformation-initiative-starts-with-a-t/ArticleStandard/Article/detail/127457—Ken Krizner.

38. www.ou.edu/deptcomm/dodjcc/groups/99A2/theories.htm.

39. sphweb.bumc.bu.edu/otlt/MPH-Modules/SB/BehavioralChangeTheories/BehavioralChangeTheories4.html.

40. web.stanford.edu/class/symbsys205/Diffusion%20of%20Innovations.htm.

41. electronicsforu.com/technology-trends/managed-leased-line-network.

42. www.who.int/healthpromotion/about/HPR%20Glossary_New%20Terms.pdf.

43. www.powershow.com/view0/6b1025-ZjE5N/Big_data_analytics_in_Healthcare_power-point_ppt_presentation.

44. Zanella A, Bui N, Castellani A, Vangelista L, Zorzi M. Internet of things for smart cities. IEEE Internet Things J. 2014;1(1):22–32.

45. Big data and analytics in healthcare overview—fueling the journey toward better outcomes, Sri Srinivasan, Global Industry Leader, Big Data & Analytics, Healthcare & Life Sciences, September 2014.

46. Raghupathi W, Raghupathi V. Big data analytics in healthcare: promise and potential. Health Inf Sci Syst. 2014;2:3. http://www.hissjournal.com/content/2/1/3.

47. Dimitrov DV. Medical internet of things and big data in healthcare. Healthc Inform Res. 2016;22(3):156–63. doi:10.4258/hir.2016.22.3.156.

48. en.wikipedia.org/wiki/Internet_of_things.

Index

© Springer Nature Singapore Pte Ltd. 2017
S.B. Bhattacharyya, *A DIY Guide to Telemedicine for Clinicians*,
DOI 10.1007/978-981-10-5305-4